D0927464

HUMANIZING HOSPITAL CARE

HUMANIZING HOSPITAL CARE

Edited by

Gerald P. Turner
Joseph Mapa

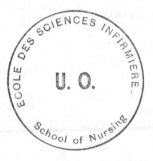

McGraw-Hill Ryerson

Toronto, Montreal, New York, St. Louis, San Francisco, Auckland, Beirut,
Bogotá, Düsseldorf, Johannesburg, Lisbon, London, Lucerne, Madrid,
Mexico, New Delhi, Panama, Paris, San Juan, São Paulo, Singapore,
Sydney, Tokyo

HUMANIZING HOSPITAL CARE

Copyright © McGraw-Hill Ryerson Limited, 1979. All rights reserved. No part
of this publication may be reproduced, stored in a retrieval system, or
transmitted, in any form, or by any means, electronic, mechanical, photocopying,
recording, or otherwise, without prior written permission of McGraw-Hill
Ryerson Limited.

ISBN 0-07-082937-3

1 2 3 4 5 6 7 8 9 10 D 8 7 6 5 4 3 2 1 0 9

Printed and bound in Canada

Canadian Cataloguing in Publication Data

Canadian Cataloguing in Publication Data

Main entry under title:

Humanizing hospital care

ISBN 0-07-082937-3

1. Hospital care - Addresses, essays, lectures.
I. Turner, Gerald P., date. II. Mapa, Joseph,
date.

RA972.H85   362.1'1   C79-094096-5

For Clare and Sheryl

'Tis remarkable, that nothing touches a man of humanity more than any instance of extraordinary delicacy in love or friendship, where a person is attentive to the smallest concerns of his friend, and is willing to sacrifice to them the most considerable interest of his own. Such delicacies have little influence on society; because they make us regard the greatest trifles. But they are the more engaging, the more minute the concern is, and are a proof of the highest merit in any one, who is capable of them. The passions are so contagious, that they pass with the greatest facility from one person to another, and produce correspondent movements in all human breasts. Where friendship appears in very signal instances, my heart catches the same passion, and is warm'd by those warm sentiments, that display themselves before me.

David Hume, *A Treatise of Human Nature*

Table of Contents

Preface

In hospital care, humanism and science must be inextricably intertwined. Although this has been emphasized throughout the ages, this fact is of sufficient importance and of contemporary necessity to be re-emphasized here. This book is a collection of some of the most outstanding contributions to the development of this understanding. The book is unique in several respects, especially in its interpretation, within an overall framework, of the various components and perspectives that form the basis of humanistic hospital care.

The subject of humanism and hospital care has an undeniable relevance for much of our thinking as health professionals, health students, and health consumers. Our objective and hope are that, by professionally exploring vital issues from a humanistic perspective, all of us may become more circumspect, more reflective about ourselves in relation to our patients, and about the relation of our professions to the larger community. Without these perspectives it may be difficult to go on with equanimity and understanding.

The book should be of interest to those members of the health profession and general public who wish to integrate and advance their knowledge of the role of humanism in health care, and their ability to apply this knowledge in the real world.

Fortunately, this topic has received extensive coverage which is supported by pertinent and considerable literature. The work already done in this field can, if properly integrated, provide valuable insight for the reader. This book attempts to do this.

Without efforts directed towards concepts and philosophies, there can be no real progress toward better serving our communities. More vital, however, is the realization that understanding is not enough. If concepts are to have significant impact on the health care of our communities, they must be applied.

For this reason we have selected a group of specific articles that we believe will be of significant value to the application of the humanistic concept in health care. The book is divided into five sections, and the themes of the materials are explained in the introductions to each of the sections. An attempt is made to provide a multi-dimensional and multi-disciplinary representation of most of the major perspectives concerning humanistic health care.

Gerald P. Turner and
Joseph Mapa

Toronto, Canada

Contributors

Bernard Barber, Department of Sociology, Barnard College of Columbia University.

E. Michael Bluestone, Graduate School of Public Administration, New York University.

Fred Davis, Department of Sociology, University of California, San Diego.

Avedis Donabedian, School of Public Health, Department of Medical Care Organization, University of Michigan.

George L. Engel, Departments of Psychiatry and Medicine, The University of Rochester, School of Medicine and Dentistry.

Theodore J. Freedman, Mount Sinai Hospital, Toronto, Canada.

Dominic S. Harveston, The Wright Institute, University of California, Berkeley.

Marie R. Haug, Department of Sociology, Case Western Reserve University.

Jan Howard, School of Medicine, University of California, San Francisco

David Hayes-Bautista, School of Public Health, University of California, Berkeley

Ivan Illich, Centre for International Documentation, Cuernavaca, Mexico.

Beatrice J. Kalisch, University of Michigan School of Nursing.

Jay L. Lebow, Dupage County Mental Health Department, Westmount, Illinois.

Judith Lorber, Department of Sociology, Brooklyn College of the City University of New York.

Hans O. Mauksch, School of Medicine, Department of Family and Community Medicine, Section of Behavioural Sciences, University of Missouri-Columbia.

Francis W. Peabody (Deceased), Harvard University Medical School.

Edmund D. Pellegrino, Yale University School of Medicine.

Clyde Pope, Health Services Research Centre, Kaiser Foundation Hospitals.

Leo G. Reeder, School of Public Health, Centre for Health Sciences, University of California, Los Angeles.

Sheryl Ruzek, Program for Women in the Health Sciences, University of California, San Francisco.

Raphella Sohier, University of Illinois Medical Centre.

Allison J. Stuart, Mount Sinai Hospital, Toronto, Canada.

Thomas S. Szasz, College of Medicine, Department of Psychiatry, State University of New York, Upstate Medical Centre, Syracuse.

Daisy L. Tagliacozzo, Department of Sociology, University of Massachusetts.

HUMANIZING HOSPITAL CARE

A Humane Ideology

Introduction

This section serves as a conceptual framework. It provides a philosophical background against which the various perspectives of humanization in health care are delineated throughout the book. The significance of the article which comprises this section is that it elucidates that the principal elements of the health care process are people. And thus, the human, the unique, the psychological, the social, the non-scientific value dimensions are by definition an essential and fundamental aspect of health care.

This is the main consideration emerging from a contemplation of this section. Everything else in health care — education, research, and administration — emanate therefrom. It points out that one of the essential qualities of the health practitioner is humanism — that is, empathy, compassion and respect for the freedom, dignity, worth and belief systems of the individual person — for the "secret of the care of the patient is in caring for the patient."

Although written fifty-two years ago, Francis Weld Peabody's classic essay "The Care of the Patient," remains poignant in its universalism and contemporary in its insights and queries. In our first selection, Dr. Peabody points out that care and cure are inexorably linked; that the art and science of medicine need each other in order to be fruitful. Early in his essay, Dr. Peabody poses the pivotal question: "Can the practitioner's art be grafted on the main trunk of the fundamental sciences in such a way that there may arise a symmetrical growth, like an expanding tree, the leaves of which shall be for the 'healing of the nations'?"

That we tend, so often, despite Peabody's insistence, to maintain the gap between caring and curing, is only indicative that the answer is not easy.

The Care of the Patient

Francis W. Peabody

It is probably fortunate that most systems of education are constantly under the fire of general criticism, for if education were left solely in the hands of teachers the chances are good that it would soon deteriorate. Medical education, however, is less likely to suffer from stagnation, for whenever the lay public stops criticizing the type of modern doctor, the medical profession itself may be counted on to stir up the stagnant pool and cleanse it of its sedimentary deposit. The most common criticism made at present by older practitioners is that young graduates have been taught a great deal about the mechanisms of disease, but very little about the practice of medicine — or, to put it more bluntly, they are too "scientific" and do not know how to take care of patients.

One is, of course, somewhat tempted to question how completely fitted for his life work the practitioner of the older generation was when he first entered it, and how much the haze of time has led him to confuse what he learned in the school of medicine with what he acquired in the harder school of experience. The indictment is a serious one, agreed upon by numerous recent graduates, who find that in the actual practice of medicine they encounter many situations which they had not been led to anticipate and which they are not prepared to meet effectively. Where there is so much smoke, there is undoubtedly a good deal of fire, and the problem for teachers and for students is to consider what they can do to extinguish whatever is left of this smoldering distrust.

The Art and Science of Medicine

To begin with, the fact must be accepted that one cannot expect to become a skillful practitioner of medicine in the four or five years allotted to the medical curriculum. Medicine is not a trade to be learned but a profession to be entered. It is an ever-widening field that requires continued study and prolonged experience in close contact with the sick. All that the medical school can hope to do is to supply the foundations on which to build. When one considers the amazing progress of science in its relation to medicine during the last thirty years, and the enormous mass of scientific material which must be made available to the modern physician, it is not surprising that the schools have tended to concern themselves more and more with this phase of the educational problem. And while they have been absorbed in the difficult task of digesting and correlating new knowledge, it has been easy to overlook the fact that the application of the

From *The Journal Of The American Medical Association,* Vol.88, March 19, 1927, 877-882. Copyright 1927, American Medical Association. By permission of the publisher.

principles of science to the diagnosis and treatment of disease is only one limited aspect of medical practice. The practice of medicine in its broadest sense includes the whole relationship of the physician with his patient. It is an art, based to an increasing extent on the medical sciences, but comprising much that still remains outside the realm of any science. The art of medicine and the science of medicine are not antagonistic but supplementary to each other. There is no more contradiction between the science of medicine and the art of medicine than between the science of aeronautics and the art of flying. Good practice presupposes an understanding of the sciences which contribute to the structure of modern medicine, but it is obvious that sound professional training should include a much broader equipment.

The problem that I wish to consider, therefore, is whether this larger view of the profession cannot be approached even under the conditions imposed by the present curriculum of the medical school. Can the practitioner's art be grafted on the main trunk of the fundamental sciences in such a way that there may arise a symmetrical growth, like an expanding tree, the leaves of which shall be for the "healing of the nations"?

The physician who speaks of patient care is naturally thinking about circumstances as they exist in the practice of medicine; but the teacher who is attempting to train medical students is immediately confronted by the fact that, even if he would, he cannot make the conditions under which he has to teach clinical medicine exactly similar to those of actual practice.

The primary difficulty is that instruction has to be carried out largely in the wards and dispensaries of hospitals rather than in the patient's home and the physician's office. Now, the essence of practicing medicine is that it is an intensely personal matter, and one of the chief differences between private practice and hospital practice is that the latter always tends to become impersonal. At first sight this may not appear to be a very vital point, but it is, as a matter of fact, the crux of the whole situation. The treatment of a disease may be entirely impersonal; the care of a patient must be completely personal. The significance of the intimate personal relationship between physician and patient cannot be too strongly emphasized, for in an extraordinarily large number of cases both diagnosis and treatment are directly dependent on it, and the failure of the young physician to establish this relationship accounts for much of his ineffectiveness in the care of patients.

HOSPITALS   Hospitals — like other institutions founded with the highest human ideals — are apt to deteriorate into dehumanized machines, and even the physician who has the patient's welfare most at heart finds that the pressure of work forces him to give most of his attention to the critically sick and to those whose diseases are a menace to the public health. In such cases he must first treat the specific disease, and then there remains little time in which to cultivate more than a superficial personal contact with the patients. Moreover, the circumstances under which the physician sees the patient are not wholly favorable to establishing the intimate personal relationship that exists in private practice, for one of the outstanding features of hospitalization is that it completely removes the patient from his accustomed environment. This may, of course, be entirely desirable, and one of the main reasons for sending a person into the hospital is to get him away from home surroundings, which, be he rich or poor, are often unfavorable for recovery; but at the same time it is equally important for the physician to know the exact character of those surroundings.

Everybody, sick or well, is affected in one way or another, consciously or subconsciously, by the material and spiritual forces that bear on his life, and especially to the sick such forces may act as powerful stimulants or depressants. When the general practitioner goes into the home of a patient, he may know the whole background of the family life from past experience; but even when he comes as a stranger he has every opportunity to find out what manner of man his patient is, and what kind of circumstances make his life. He gets a hint of financial anxiety or of domestic incompatibility; he may find himself confronted by a querulous, exacting, self-centered patient, or by a gentle invalid overawed by a dominating family; as he appreciates how these circumstances are affecting the patient he dispenses sympathy, encouragement, or discipline. What is spoken of as a "clinical picture" is not just a photograph of a man sick in bed; it is an impressionistic painting of the patient surrounded by his home, his work, his relations, his friends, his joys, sorrows, hopes, and fears. Now, all of this background of sickness which bears so strongly on the symptomatology is liable to be lost sight of in the hospital. (I say "liable to" because it is not by any means always lost sight of and because I believe that by making a constant and conscious effort one can almost always bring it out into its proper perspective.) The difficulty is that in the hospital one gets into the habit of using the oil immersion lens instead of the low power, and focuses too intently on the center of the field.

When a patient enters a hospital, the first thing that commonly happens to him is that he loses his personal identity. He is generally referred to not as Henry Jones, but as "that case of mitral stenosis in the second bed on the left." There are plenty of reasons why this is so, and the point is, in itself, relatively unimportant; but the trouble is that it leads more or less directly to the patient being treated as a case of mitral stenosis, and not as a sick man. The disease is treated, but Henry Jones, lying awake nights while he worries about his wife and children, represents a problem that is much more complex than the pathologic physiology of mitral stenosis, and he is apt to improve very slowly unless a discerning intern discovers why it is that even large doses of digitalis fail to slow his heart rate. Henry happens to have heart disease, but he is not disturbed so much by dyspnea as he is by anxiety for the future. A talk with an understanding physician who tries to make the situation clear to him, and then gets the social service worker to find a suitable occupation, does more to straighten him out than a book full of drugs and diets. Henry has an excellent example of a certain type of heart disease, and he is glad that all the staff find him interesting, for it makes him feel that they will do the best they can to cure him; but just because he is an interesting case he does not cease to be a human being with very human hopes and fears. Sickness produces an abnormally sensitive emotional state in almost everyone, and in many cases the emotional state repercusses, as it were, on the organic disease. The pneumonia would probably run its course in a week, regardless of treatment, but the experienced physician knows that by quieting the cough, getting the patient to sleep, and giving a bit of encouragement, he can save his patient's strength and lift him through many distressing hours. The institutional eye tends to become focused on the lung, and it forgets that the lung is only one part of the body.

SYMPTOMS WITHOUT ORGANIC CAUSES   But if teachers and students are inclined to take a limited point of view even toward interesting cases of organic disease, they fall into much more serious error in their attitude toward a large group of patients who do not show objective, organic pathologic conditions, and who are generally spoken of as having "nothing the matter with them." Up to a certain point these patients will command attention as long as the physicians think there is a diagnostic problem, but as soon as the physician has assured himself that they do not have an organic disease, he passes over them lightly.

Take the case of a young woman, for instance, who entered the hospital with a history of nausea and discomfort in the upper part of the abdomen after eating. Mrs. Brown had "suffered many things of many physicians." Each of them gave her a tonic and limited her diet. She stopped eating everything that any of her physicians advised her to omit, and is now living on a little milk with a few crackers, but her symptoms persist. The history suggests a possible gastric ulcer or gallstones, and with a proper desire to study the case thoroughly, she is given a test meal, gastric analysis, and duodenal intubation; roentgen-ray examinations are made of the gastrointestinal tract and gallbladder. All of these diagnostic methods give negative results; that is, they do not show evidence of any structural change. The case immediately becomes much less interesting than if it had turned out to be a gastric ulcer with atypical symptoms. The visiting physician walks by and says, "Well, there's nothing the matter with her." The clinical clerk says, "I did an awful lot of work on that case and it turned out to be nothing at all." The intern, who wants to clear out the ward so as to make room for some interesting cases, says, "Mrs. Brown, you can send for your clothes and go home tomorrow. There really is nothing the matter with you, and fortunately you have not got any of the serious trouble we suspected. We have used all the most modern and scientific methods and we find that there is no reason why you should not eat anything you want to. I will give you a tonic to take when you go home." Same story, same colored medicine! Mrs. Brown goes home, somewhat better for her rest in new surroundings, thinking that nurses are kind and physicians are pleasant, but that they do not seem to know much about the sort of medicine that will touch her trouble. She takes up her life and the symptoms return — and then she tries chiropractic, or perhaps Christian Science.

It is rather fashionable to say that the modern physician has become "too scientific." Now, was it too scientific, with all the stomach tubes and blood counts and roentgen-ray examinations? Not at all. Mrs. Brown's symptoms might have been due to a gastric ulcer or to gallstones, and after such a long course it was only proper to use every method that might help to clear the diagnosis. Was it, perhaps, not scientific enough? The popular conception of a scientist as a man who works in a laboratory and who uses instruments of precision is as inaccurate as it is superficial, for a scientist is known, not by his technical processes, but by his intellectual processes; and the essence of the scientific method of thought is that it proceeds in an orderly manner toward establishing a truth. The chief criticism to be made of the way Mrs. Brown's case was handled is that the staff was contented with a half-truth. The investigation of the patient was decidedly unscientific in that it stopped short of even an attempt to determine the real cause of the symptoms. As soon as organic disease could be excluded the whole problem was given up, but the symptoms persisted. Speaking candidly, the case was a medical failure in spite of the fact that the patient went home with the assurance that there was "nothing the matter" with her.

A good many "Mrs. Browns," male and female, come to hospitals, and a great many more go to private physicians. They are all characterized by the presence of symptoms that cannot be accounted for by organic disease, and they are all liable to be told that they have "nothing the matter" with them. Now, my own experience as a hospital physician has been rather long and varied, and I have always found that, from my point of view, hospitals are particularly interesting and cheerful places; but I am fairly certain that, except for a few people who want to get in out of the cold, there are not many people who become hospital patients unless there is something the matter with them. And, by the same token, I doubt whether there are many people, except for those who would rather go to the physician than go to the theater, who spend their money on visiting private physicians unless there is something the matter with them. In the hospital and in private practice, however, one finds this same type of patient, and many physicians whom I have questioned agree that, excluding cases of acute infection, approximately half of their patients complained of symptoms for which an adequate organic cause could not be discovered. Numerically, then, these patients constitute a large group, and their fees go a long way toward spreading butter on the doctor's bread. Medically speaking, they are not serious cases as regards prospective death, but they are often extremely serious as regards prospective life. Their symptoms will rarely prove fatal, but their lives will be long and miserable, and they may end by nearly exhausting their families and friends. Death is not the worst thing in the world, and to help a man have a happy and useful career may be more of a service than saving life.

What is the matter with all these patients? Technically, most of them come under the broad heading of the "psychoneurotics"; but for practical purposes many of them may be regarded as patients whose subjective symptoms are due to disturbances of the physiologic activity of one or more organs or systems. These symptoms may depend on an increase or a decrease of a normal function, on an abnormality of function, or merely on the subjects becoming conscious of wholly normal function that normally goes on unnoticed; and this last conception indicates that there is a close relation between the appearance of the symptoms and the threshold of the patient's nervous reactions. The ultimate causes of these disturbances are to be found not in any gross structural changes of the organs involved, but rather in nervous influences emanating from the emotional or intellectual life which, directly or indirectly, affect in one way or another organs that are under either voluntary or involuntary control.

All of you have had experiences that have brought home the way in which emotional reactions affect organic functions. Some of you have been nauseated while anxiously waiting for an important examination to begin, and a few may even have vomited; others have been seized by an attack of diarrhea under the same circumstances. Some of you have had polyuria before making a speech, and others have felt thumping extrasystoles or a pounding tachycardia before a football game. Some have noticed rapid shallow breathing when listening to a piece of bad news, and others know the type of occipital headache, with pain down the muscles of the back of the neck, that comes from nervous anxiety and fatigue.

These are all simple examples of the way that emotional reactions may upset the normal functioning of an organ. Vomiting and diarrhea are due to abnormalities of the motor function of the gastrointestinal tract — one to the production of an active reversed peristalsis of the stomach and a relaxation of the cardia sphincter, the other to hyperperistalsis of the large intestine. The polyuria is caused by vasomotor changes that take place in the peripheral vessels in blushing and blanching of the skin, and in addition there are quite possibly associated changes in the rate of blood flow and in blood pressure. Tachycardia and extrasystoles indicate that not only the rate but also the rhythm of the heart is under a nervous control that can be demonstrated in the intact human being as well as in the laboratory animal. The ventilatory function of the respiration is extraordinarily subject to nervous influences; so much so, in fact, that the study of respiration in man is associated with peculiar difficulties. Rate, depth, and rhythm of breathing are easily upset by even minor stimuli, and in extreme cases the disturbance in total ventilation is sometimes so great that gaseous exchange becomes affected. Thus, I remember an emotional young woman who developed a respiratory neurosis with deep and rapid breathing and expired so much carbon dioxide that the symptoms of tetany ensued.

The explanation of the occipital headaches and of so many pains in the muscles of the back is not entirely clear, but they appear to be associated with changes in muscular tone or with prolonged states of contraction.

There is certainly a very intimate correlation between mental tenseness and muscular tenseness, and whatever methods are used to produce mental relaxation will usually cause muscular relaxation, together with relief of this type of pain. A similar condition is found in so-called writers' cramp, in which the painful muscles of the hand result not from manual work but from mental work.

One might go much further, but these few illustrations will suffice to recall the infinite number of ways in which physiologic functions may be upset by emotional stimuli, and the manner in which the resulting disturbances of function manifest themselves as symptoms. These symptoms, although obviously not due to anatomic changes, may nevertheless be very disturbing and distressing, and there is nothing imaginary about them. Emotional vomiting is just as real as the vomiting due to pyloric obstruction, and so-called nervous headaches may be as painful as headaches resulting from a brain tumor. Moreover, it must be remembered that symptoms based on functional disturbances may be present in a patient who has, at the same time, organic disease, and in such cases the determination of the causes of the different symptoms may be an extremely difficult matter. Everyone accepts the relationship between the common function symptoms and nervous reactions, for convincing evidence is to be found in the fact that under ordinary circumstances the symptoms disappear just as soon as the emotional cause has passed. But what happens if the cause does not pass away? What if, instead of having to face a single three-hour examination, one has to face a life of being constantly ill? The emotional stimulus persists and continues to produce the disturbances of function. As with all nervous reactions, the longer the process goes on, or the more frequently it goes on, the easier it is for it to continue. The unusual nervous track becomes an established path. After a time, the symptom and the subjective discomfort that it produces come to occupy the center of the picture, and the causative factors recede into a hazy background. The patient no longer thinks, "I cannot stand this life," but he says aloud, "I cannot stand this nausea and vomiting. I must go to see a stomach specialist."

Quite possibly your comment on this will be that the symptoms of such "neurotic" patients are well known, and they ought to go to a neurologist or a psychiatrist and not to an internist or a general practitioner. In an era of internal medicine, however, which takes pride in the fact that it concerns itself with the functional capacity of organs rather than with mere structural changes, and which has developed so many "functional tests" for kidneys, heart, and liver, is it not rather narrow-minded to limit one's interest to those disturbances of function which are based on anatomic abnormalities?

There are other reasons, too, why most of these "functional" cases belong to the field of general medicine. In the first place, the differential diagnosis between organic disease and pure functional disturbance is often extremely difficult, and it needs the broad training in the use of general clinical and laboratory methods which forms the equipment of the internist. Diagnosis is the first step in treatment. In the second place, the patients themselves frequently prefer to go to a medical practitioner rather than to a psychiatrist, and in the long run it is probably better for them to get straightened out without having what they often consider the stigma of having been "nervous" cases. A limited number, it is true, are so refractory or so complex that the aid of the psychiatrist must be sought, but the majority can be helped by the internist without highly specialized psychologic technic, if he will appreciate the significance of functional disturbances and interest himself in their treatment. The physician who does take these cases seriously — one might say scientifically — has the great satisfaction of seeing some of his patients get well, not as the result of drugs or as the result of the disease having run its course, but as the result of his own individual efforts.

Here, then, is a great group of patients in which it is not the disease but the man or the woman who needs to be treated. In general, hospital practice physicians are so busy with the critically sick, and in clinical teaching they are so concerned with training students in physical diagnosis and attempting to show them all types of organic disease, that they do not pay as much attention as they should to the functional disorders. Many a student enters upon his career having hardly heard of them except in his course in psychiatry, and without the faintest conception of how large a part they will play in his future practice. At best, his method of treatment is apt to be a cheerful reassurance combined with a placebo. The successful diagnosis and treatment of these patients, however, depend almost entirely upon establishing that intimate personal contact between physician and patient which forms the basis of private practice. Without this, it is virtually impossible for the physician to get an idea of the problems and troubles that lie behind so many functional disorders. If students are to obtain any insight into this field of medicine, they must also be given opportunities to build up the same type of personal relationship with their patients.

TEACHING CONDITIONS   Is there, then, anything inherent in the conditions of clinical teaching in a general hospital that makes this impossible? Can you form a personal relationship in an impersonal institution? Can you accept the fact that your patient is entirely removed from his natural environment and then reconstruct the background of environment from the history, the family, a visit to the home or workshop, and from the information obtained by the social service worker? And while you are building up this environmental background, can you enter into the same personal relationship that you ought to have in private practice? If you can do all this, and I know from experience that you can, then the study of medicine in the hospital actually becomes the practice of medicine, and the treatment of disease immediately takes its proper place in the larger problem of caring for the patient.

When a patient goes to a physician he usually has confidence that the physician is the best, or at least the best available, person to help him with his trouble. He relies on the physician as a sympathetic adviser and a wise professional counselor. When a patient goes to a hospital he has confidence in the reputation of the institution, but it is hardly necessary to add that he also hopes to come into contact with some individual who personifies the institution and will also take a human interest in him. It is obvious that the first physician to see the patient is in the strategic position — and in hospitals all students can have the satisfaction of being regarded as physicians.

For example, consider the poor man who has just been jolted to the hospital in an ambulance. A string of questions about himself and his family has been fired at him, his valuables and even his clothes have been taken away from him, and he is wheeled into the ward on a truck, miserable, scared, defenseless, and, in his nakedness, unable to run away. He is lifted into a bed, becomes conscious of the fact that he is the center of interest in the ward, wishes that he had stayed at home among friends, and, just as he is beginning to take stock of his surroundings, finds that a thermometer is being stuck under his tongue. It is all strange and new, and he wonders what is going to happen next. The next thing that does happen is that a man in a long white coat sits down by his bedside, and starts to talk to him.

Now, it happens that according to our system of clinical instruction that man is usually a medical student. Do you see what an opportunity you have? The foundation of your whole relation with that patient is laid in those first few minutes of contact, just as happens in private practice. Here is a worried, lonely, suffering man, and if you begin by approaching him with sympathy, tact, and consideration, you get his confidence and he becomes *your* patient. Interns and visiting physicians may come and go, and the hierarchy gives them a precedence; but if you make the most of your opportunities he will regard you as his personal physician, and all the rest as mere consultants. Of course, you must not drop him after you have taken the history and made your physical examination. Once your relationship with him has been established, you must foster it by every means. Watch his condition closely and he will see that you are alert professionally. Make time to have little talks with him — and these talks need not always be about his symptoms. Remember that you want to know him as a man, and this means you must know about his family and friends, his work and his play. What kind of person is he — cheerful, depressed, introspective, careless, conscientious, mentally keen or dull? Look out for all the little incidental things that you can do for his comfort. These, too, are a part of "caring for the patient." Some of them will fall technically into the field of "nursing," but you will always be profoundly grateful for any nursing technic that you have acquired. It is worth your while to get the nurse to teach you the right way to feed a patient, change the bed, or give a bed pan. Do you know the practical tricks that make a dyspneic patient comfortable? Assume some responsibility for these apparently minor points and you will find that it is when you are doing some such friendly service, rather than when you are a formal questioner, that the patient suddenly starts to unburden himself, and a flood of light is thrown on the situation.

Meantime, of course, you will have been active along strictly medical lines, and by the time your clinical and laboratory examinations are completed you will be surprised to see how intimately you know your patient, not only as an interesting case but also as a sick human being. Everything you have picked up about him will be of value in handling the situation later. Suppose, for instance, you find conclusive evidence that his symptoms are due to organic disease: say, to a gastric ulcer. As soon as you face the problem of laying out his regimen you find that it is one thing to write an examination paper on treating gastric ulcer and quite another thing to treat John Smith, who happens to have a gastric ulcer. You want to begin by giving him rest in bed and a special diet for eight weeks. Rest means both nervous and physical rest. Can he get it best at home or in the hospital? What are the conditions at home? If you keep him in the hospital, it is probably good for him to see certain people, and bad for him to see others. He has business problems that must be considered. What kind of compromise can you make on them? How about the financial implications of eight weeks in bed followed by a period of convalescence? Is it, on the whole, wiser to try a strict regimen for a shorter period, and, if he does not improve, take up the question of operation sooner than is in general advisable? These and many similar problems arise in the course of treating almost every patient, and they have to be considered, not from the abstract point of view of treating the disease, but from the concrete point of view of caring for the individual.

Suppose, on the other hand, that all your clinical and laboratory examinations turn out entirely negative as far as revealing any evidence of organic disease is concerned. Then you are in the difficult position of not having discovered the explanation of the patient's symptoms. You have merely assured yourself that certain conditions are not present. Of course, the first thing you have to consider is whether these symptoms are the result of organic disease in such an early stage that you cannot definitely recognize it. This problem is often extremely perplexing, requiring great clinical experience for its solution, and often you will be forced to fall back on time in which to watch developments. If, however, you finally exclude recognizable organic disease, and the probability of early or very slight organic disease, it becomes necessary to consider whether the symptomatology may be due to a functional disorder which is caused by nervous or emotional influences. You know a good deal about the personal life of your patient by this time, but perhaps there is nothing that stands out as an obvious etiologic factor, and it becomes necessary to sit down for a long intimate talk with him to discover what has remained hidden.

EMOTIONAL CONDITIONS   Sometimes it is well to explain to the patient, by obvious examples, how it is that emotional states may bring about symptoms similar to his own, so that he will understand what you are driving at and will cooperate with you. Often the best way is to go back to the very beginning and try to find out the circumstances of the patient's life at the time the symptoms first began. The association between symptoms and cause may have been simpler and more direct at the onset, at least in the patient's mind, for as time goes on, and the symptoms become more pronounced and distressing, there is a natural tendency for the symptoms to occupy so much of the foreground of the picture that the background is completely obliterated. Sorrow, disappointment, anxiety, self-distrust, thwarted ideals or ambitions in social, business, or personal life, and particularly what are called maladaptations to these conditions — these are among the most common and simplest factors that initiate and perpetuate the functional disturbances.

Perhaps you will find that the digestive disturbances began at the time the patient was in serious financial difficulties, and that they have recurred whenever he is worried about money matters. Or you may find that ten years ago a physician told the patient he had heart disease, cautioning him "not to worry about it." For ten years the patient has never mentioned the subject, but he has avoided every exertion, and has lived with the idea that sudden death was in store for him. You will find that physicians, by wrong diagnoses and ill-considered statements, are responsible for many wrecked lives, and you will discover that it is much easier to make a wrong diagnosis than it is to "unmake" it. Or, again, you may find that the pain in this woman's back made its appearance when she first felt her domestic unhappiness, and that this man's headaches have been associated, not with long hours of work, but with a constant depression due to unfulfilled ambitions. The causes are manifold and the manifestations protean. Sometimes the mechanism of cause and effect is obvious; sometimes it becomes apparent only after a very tangled skein has been unraveled.

If the establishment of an intimate personal relationship is necessary in diagnosing functional disturbances, it becomes doubly necessary in their treatment. Unless there is complete confidence in the sympathetic understanding of the physician as well as in his professional skill, very little can be accomplished; assuming that you have been able to get close enough to the patient to discover the cause of the trouble, you will find that a general hospital is not at all an impossible place for treating functional disturbances. The hospital has, indeed, the advantage that the entire reputation of the institution, and all that it represents in the way of facilities for diagnosis and treatment, help to enhance the confidence which the patient has in the individual physician who represents it. This gives the very young physician a hold on his patients that he could scarcely hope to have without its support. Another advantage is that hospital patients are removed from their usual environment, for treating functional disturbances is often easier when patients are away from friends, relatives, home, work, and, indeed, everything that is associated with their daily life. It is true that in a public ward one cannot obtain complete isolation in the sense that this is a part of the Weir Mitchell treatment, but the main object is accomplished if one has obtained the psychologic effect of isolation which comes with an entirely new and unaccustomed atmosphere. The conditions, therefore, under which you as students come into contact with patients with functional disturbances are not wholly unfavorable, and with very little effort they can be made to simulate closely the conditions in private practice.

It is not my purpose, however, to go into a discussion of the methods of treating functional disturbances, and I have dwelled on the subject only because these cases illustrate so clearly the vital importance of the personal relationship between physician and patient in the practice of medicine. In all your patients whose symptoms are of functional origin, the whole problem of diagnosis and treatment depends on your insight into the patient's character and personal life, and in every case of organic disease there are complex interactions between the pathologic processes and the intellectual processes which you must appreciate and consider if you would be a wise clinician. There are moments, of course, in cases of serious illness when you will think solely of the disease and its treatment; but when the corner is turned and the immediate crisis is passed, you must give your attention to the patient. Disease in man is never exactly the same as disease in an experimental animal, for in man the disease at once affects and is affected by what we call the emotional life. Thus, the physician who attempts to take care of a patient while he neglects this factor is as unscientific as the investigator who neglects to control all the conditions that may affect his experiment. The good physician knows his patients through and through, and his knowledge is bought dearly. Time, sympathy, and understanding must be lavishly dispensed, but the reward is to be found in that personal bond which forms the greatest satisfaction of the practice of medicine. One of the essential qualities of the clinician is interest in humanity, for the secret of the care of the patient is in caring *for* the patient.

Disappointed Idealism

Introduction

The articles in this section suggest that no single factor will explain the inherent dehumanizing tendencies of today's pattern of health care. It is a multi-causal development, with some factors immediate; others profound and complex. These articles are only a sample portion of the many analyses being conducted by social and behavioural scientists and health practitioners; but they illustrate the scope and variety of reasons for the dehumanization process.

The contemporary discontent with the dehumanization tendencies in health care — which many may lament, even though it is difficult if not impossible to deny — exists because people care. This in itself, gives us cause for hope for "it reflects not cynicism but disappointed idealism."

Technology, specialization, institutionalization, professionalism, bureaucratization, routinization, social evolution, and emphasis on efficiency, have tended to submerge the humanistic aspect of health care — an ideal which is still relevant and attainable. Understanding the causes of this contemporary phenomenon is of paramount importance towards the fulfillment of this ideal. Remedies depend for their effectiveness on the identification and relationships of causal factors.

The first article by Jan Howard et al, "Humanizing Health Care: The Implications of Technology, Centralization, and Self-Care" presents a penetrating and systematic analysis of technology and centralization as crucial sources of dehumanization and suggests strategies for change; including the concept of Self-Help Care which "has emerged to fill serious gaps in service and to offer alternatives to forms of traditional care which are viewed as ineffective, inappropriate, or too expensive."

In our second article, "The Implications of 'Failure of Communication' in Hospitals," Dr. E. Michael Bluestone concentrates on the failure of communications between the patient and the health practitioner in an institutional setting. Bluestone examines the meaning of communication and lack of communication in a hospital and indicates that "in one way or another, this (communication) failure, aggravates the mental or physical condition of the patient — after he was admitted in the hope that, by words as well as deeds, he would be sheltered from all harm." In other words, failure of communication with the patients is one factor which threatens the hospital's "very humane ideology."

In our third selection Beatrice J. Kalisch, in "Of Half Gods and Mortals:

Aesculapian Authority" illuminates the "dynamics of the patient-physician relationship and explores a phenomenon labeled aesculapian authority, that usually goes unnoticed but nonetheless plays a highly significant role in the health delivery system." Professor Kalisch points out that the pervasiveness of this medical (and nursing) model — which stems from a three pronged power base: the physician's expertise, the patient's faith in him and the belief that he has almost mystical powers — accounts, to a large extent, for the depersonalization which patients so often experience in the health system.

The authority of the physician, a phenomenon which Kalisch has labelled "aesculapian authority" has become a subject of increasing interest to social and behavioural scientists. In our final selection of this section, "The Erosion of Professional Authority: A Cross Cultural Inquiry in the Case of the Physician," Marie R. Haug expands this topic by examining the extent to which the erosion of professional authority observed in the United States is also occurring in the United Kingdom and the U.S.S.R., in the case of the primary physician. Education of the patient emerged as a critical factor in eroding physician authority in both countries.

Humanizing Health Care:
The Implications of Technology,
Centralization and Self-Care

Jan Howard, Fred Davis, Clyde Pope, and Sheryl Ruzek

The committee on the humanization of health care conducted a series of pilot studies to identify dehumanizing practices in medicine and possible modes of change. The work of the group was enhanced by the participation of forty health professionals and behavioural scientists in the Symposium on Humanizing Health Care held in December, 1972. It focused on the concept, causes, and consequences of dehumanization and on alternatives to current styles of practice. All the papers presented at the conference, commentaries on them, and several additional articles on research strategies were incorporated in the book *Humanizing Health Care*, edited by Jan Howard and Anselm Strauss and published by John Wiley and Sons in the summer of 1975.[22]

Since the Symposium, members of the committee have explored in greater depth a number of the issues it raised. Fred Davis has investigated the dehumanizing consequences of bureaucratic medicine and the ingenious attempts of patients to "beat the system" and force a positive response to their wants and needs. Sheryl Ruzek has systematically studied women's health collectives, clinics, and self-help gynecology groups on the West Coast and their potential for humanizing routine gynecologic care.[39] Julius Roth has outlined a handbook for consumers that would describe the real workings of medical systems and help patients deal with them more effectively and appropriately, while preserving their dignity as human beings.

Mary Lee Ingbar conducted a pilot study of the costs and benefits of different approaches to patients in a cardiac clinic. She focused on factors affecting therapeutic compliance and concluded that a special staff person should be assigned the task of monitoring and facilitating compliance. Clyde Pope expanded his research in a prepaid medical plan to include assessments of patient satisfaction with the social context of care. Tom Scheff initiated a study of the components of provider affect (warmth and coldness) as conveyed to patients.[23] Jan Howard is presently exploring humanizing and dehumanizing features of informed consent procedures in medical experiments that involve randomization.*

Out of the myriad of issues that have stimulated the work of the committee, this article addresses three topics that have significant implications for public and private policy making in the health field. We

From *Medical Care*, Vol. XV, No. 5, Supplement, May 1977. By permission of the authors and publisher.

focus on the humanizing and dehumanizing impact of technology, centralization, and self care; and we suggest strategies for change. Jan Howard is responsible for the section on technology. Fred Davis and Clyde Pope contributed the material on centralization, and Sheryl Ruzek is responsible for the section on self help. Recommendations appear at the end of each section and reflect the views of the contributor. Before we discuss humanization and dehumanization as dependent variables, we take a closer look at the concepts themselves.

A Conceptual Formulation

In her review of the health-care literature, Dr. Howard identified many connotations of dehumanization[19] which can be grouped into five categories[18]: the perception of people as objects ("thinging"); the instrumental use and exploitation of patients and providers; coldness and indifference in social interaction; the repression and limitation of human freedom (loss of options); and social ostracism and alienation. Actual definitions of dehumanization are rare and general in scope. Thus, David Vail views it as a "loss of human attributes,"[44] and Charles Lewis defines it as a "loss of dignity."[31] Taking her cue from Lewis, Dr. Howard has defined humanized care as "care that enhances the dignity and autonomy of patients and health professionals alike."[21]

Synonyms for dehumanization may be used such as Erving Goffman's "ritual mortification,"[13] or the popular but vague concept of "man's inhumanity to man."[40] In most writings, dehumanization and depersonalization are used interchangeably, but some scholars distinguish between them. Thus, Howard Leventhal defines depersonalization as "the splitting of the psychological and physical self" and dehumanization as "the feeling that one is isolated from others and regarded as a thing rather than a person."* David Hayes-Bautista uses personalization-depersonalization to signify the relative number of human providers participating in care and humanization-dehumanization to describe the relative degree of humanism practiced by those in attendance.[18]

In the volume she edits, Dr. Howard proposes eight necessary and sufficient conditions for humanized care.[18],[19] Three can be considered cognitive or perceptual; three are structural; and two are affective or emotional. Patients must be perceived as *unique and irreplaceable whole persons inherently worthy* of the caretaker's concern. To the extent of their capacity, they should *share in decisions* affecting their care, and their relations with providers should be *equalitarian or reciprocal,* not deferential or patronizing. Within the limits imposed by physical constraints and social mandates, patients should function as *autonomous persons* who have the right to control their own destinies. And they should be treated with *empathy and warmth* (positive affect) by their caretakers.

---

*These definitions were taken from an earlier draft of Howard Leventhal's "The Consequences of Depersonalization during Illness and Treatment: An Information Processing Model."[29]

According to Dr. Howard, most if not all the conditions necessary for the humanization of patients apply to the humanization of health professionals. They, too, are unique inherently worthy whole persons who deserve reasonable degrees of freedom and the right and responsibility to participate in decisions affecting their lives. They need to be treated with sympathy and warmth by colleagues and patients alike. And in spite of the service ethic, they must not be exploited as servants. Interactions with colleagues and supervisors should be based on principles of equalitarianism — at least the mutual acknowledgment that the relationships are human to human.

Implications of Technology

In analyzing humanized or dehumanized care as a concept, cause, consequence, or condition in need of change, it is necessary to consider the implications of the technological revolution in medicine.[43] By *technology* we mean the *tools* of the health-care trades and the *acumen* of those who apply them.

Just as the industrial revolution was blamed for much of the dehumanization accompanying capitalism, medical technology has been labeled a major cause of the dehumanization in modern health care.[11, 32, 34] Yet, the manifest purpose of medical tools and knowledge is clearly humanistic — to prolong life, to relieve pain and suffering, and to increase social functioning.

We contend that the technologies of the health-care industry can be humanizing or dehumanizing depending on how and for whom they are applied, the ideologies associated with their development and use, the structure of human relations involved, and the nature of alternative strategies that their use supersedes.

Advances in technology can be liberating forces if they increase the quantity, quality, and variety of options available to patients and practitioners.[26] When medical tools and skills keep people alive and well, they obviously expand the boundaries of freedom. And the greater the number and diversity of relevant tools and procedures, the greater the therapeutic alternatives open to patients. Since all human beings are unique, increasing the range of options should help maximize the fit between treatment and need.

Improvising on this theme, Eliot Freidson has proposed that patients should have the option of turning to an impersonal computer to diagnose their ailments and recommend therapy.[9] Although Freidson recognizes the limits of such a computer in dealing with the vast spectrum of human problems, his illustration suggests that not every sick person wants or needs a human therapist and that the state of technology permits alternative choices.

The hardware of health care includes machines which reduce the drudgery of work. Where they eliminate dirty work (laundry) and scut work (billing), they humanize health workers by upgrading their tasks and freeing them for more satisfying activities.

Similarly, the telephone and television can be liberating technologies by enabling providers and patients to contact and consult each other quickly and spontaneously without unnecessary time, effort, and money.[27]

By enhancing man's capacity to store and retrieve information, technology can enlarge the scope and breadth of human relations.[8] Clinical and background data supplied by a computer can transform seemingly anonymous patients into familiar whole persons to whom the provider can relate as a friend.

In light of its humanizing potential, why is technology so often considered a crucial source of dehumanization? Four ideas are relevant.

1. *Technology as a Scapegoat.*   Technology is frequently the scapegoat for social institutions, ideologies, and habits which encourage dehumanization. The tools and skills of health professionals may be falsely accused of depersonalizing patients when at most they are spurious variables. For example, a group of specialists may treat patients with cold detachment — not because the physicians have superior knowledge and hardware at their disposal but because they have "cold" personalities or because they were taught that emotional distance is the *sine qua non* of practical ethics.[35]

2. *Technology as an Indirect Source of Dehumanization.*   The implementation of technology can aggravate dehumanizing tendencies and processes already present in society. And, thus, technology might be considered an indirect rather than proximate cause of dehumanization.

Instead of increasing the available options, the impact of technology on the goals, ideologies, and authority structures of relevant social systems may decrease human freedom. In this regard Jack Geiger speaks of the "tyranny of technology" — "the idea that every scientific or technological advance is synonomous with 'progress' and must be applied."[11] This ideology is not inherent in technology. It stems from the interplay of beliefs, values, and goals in the larger society and those in the sub-society of health providers. The combined thrust of the public's demand (or hope) for a cure, the professional's commitment to respond with a visible product, and the businessman's quest for profit produce and sustain the tyranny of technology. The huge costs of discovering and developing new drugs and high-powered machines mandate their use to justify and offset the capital investment.[41]

Few policy makers attempt to compare the net value of capabilities such as renal dialysis with alternative strategies (preventive medicine or primary care) that might have a greater overall impact on the nation's health.[5] In essence, the technological imperative constricts human choice by placing undue emphasis on technological solutions to medical and social problems, undermining efforts to rationally determine priorities among the widest variety of relevant possibilities.†

---

†The line between technological and nontechnological approaches is somewhat vague, but for heuristic purposes we would regard efforts to raise the standard of living of the poor, to curtail cigarette advertising, and to enact national health insurance to be essentially nontechnological approaches.

The inclination of health professionals to exaggerate the value of "hard" therapies constrains the use of person to person approaches in health care. In the not-so-distant past, the professional's primary instrument of healing was his or her own self, laying on hands and providing tender loving care.[31] TLC is now regarded by many practitioners as placebo therapy of last resort to be prescribed when drugs, surgery, radiation, organ implants, and organ substitutes are obviously inappropriate or fail. Yet, these technologies are frequently of dubious value, or of no value, in treating the vast spectrum of social-psychological illnesses such as alcoholism, drug addiction, sexual aberrations, mental disorders, and the emotional overlay accompanying most diseases.

In dealing with many of these problems, person-to-person therapies involving insight, caring, and concern are often of greater use than the harder technologies. But the personal approaches tend to be dismissed as second-rate treatments to be provided by second-rate practitioners or lay therapists with little or no training at all. This attitude decreases therapeutic options, and pressures practitioners to prescribe the "harder" remedies, sometimes substituting one form of technological dependency for another, as in methadone programs.[28]

Advances in medical technology can expand the choices of patients by prolonging their lives. But the option to live may be an empty alternative to dying if it fails to improve the quality of life.[12] Furthermore, legal precedents as well as public and professional ethics restrain patients and their guardians from choosing death.[33] Consenting to respirators, incubators, dialysis, or chemotherapy may be a response to social demands, not an act of free will. And to stay alive in name only is to endure permanent dependency without dignity.

The existence of a medical technology does not guarantee that everyone who might benefit from its use has a chance to use it.[4] Access is generally at the discretion of the medical profession and those who exchange products or services for compensation (hospitals, pharmacies, supply houses). High-priced technologies (and the newer ones tend to be relatively expensive) are seldom universally available.

Other factors equal, the greater the usefulness of the technology, the greater the deprivation suffered by those without access. Thus, the introduction of an effective but expensive diagnostic or therapeutic tool could exacerbate an existing morbidity or mortality differential between high and low socioeconomic groups if that disparity were already unfavorable to the poor.[20] Since health affects other life chances, the aggravation of disparities in health can aggravate other disparities such as those in income, leading to a vicious circle of relative deprivations.

When effective new technologies appear, they gradually replace less useful tools. In the process, the choices of the disadvantaged may be reduced to zero if they cannot afford the newer therapies and the cheaper more anitquated ones are no longer prescribed by practitioners, or perhaps are no longer available.

To take full advantage of the options offered by technology, patients must share in medical knowledge. They need to understand what therapies are available and the probable risks and benefits. They must also be free of coercion in evaluating and selecting regimens. But many factors restrain practitioners from sharing their knowledge and skills with consumers of care. For humanistic reasons they may hesitate to tell patients the whole truth, especially when the prognosis is pessimistic and the patient's psychological state can affect the outcome or when certain risks have very low probabilities and knowledge of the unlikely will only scare the patient. Furthermore, many laymen have difficulty understanding medical information, and others verbally resist being appraised of the facts.

However, even when patients want information, whether threatening or nonthreatening, health professionals may be reluctant to respond because having a monopoly of knowledge enhances their power and prestige, and secrecy can be protective.[10] Where the norms of health providers and their guildlike associations constrain the sharing of knowledge with patients, those who are ill and their guardians are forced to defer rather blindly to the recommendations of caretakers, who tend to be biased in their choices.[36]

Deferring to the judgment of health professionals may be formalized through informed consent procedures, which temporarily bestow on providers the patient's power of choice. Even when full disclosure is the practitioner's intent, these procedures are likely to be ritualized. To appropriately inform patients of the possible risks and benefits of alternative therapies is a time-consuming process that many professionals delegate, truncate, or avoid. The constriction of information to patients may be justified for a number of reasons; but in itself it constitutes a form of coercion that is frequently reinforced by friendly or unfriendly persuasion.

The power that comes from scientific acumen and its aura is abused if it forces patients unwillingly or reluctantly into a posture of consent. When coercion occurs in the context of human experimentation,[14] it is even more vulnerable to criticism than pressures on patients to participate in tested therapies.

3. *Technology as the Direct Dehumanizing Agent.*   Some medical tools and procedures have direct and unavoidable dehumanizing consequences for patients and providers of care. These effects must be evaluated by decision makers in determining the pros and cons of utilization and possible ways to reduce and offset undesirable by-products of the dehumanization.

Jack Geiger argues that over the course of the last century, biological science has become increasingly reductionist in its view of man, fragmenting the whole person into parts and problems and converting human beings into "things," through objectification.[11] The particular perspective of modern science must be considered a dimension of technology per se. And the geometric escalation in medical tools and knowledge necessitate a division of labor which results in specialization and fragmentation.

According to Geiger, teaching about the whole man and comprehensive care has tended to have much less scientific content than physiology, biochemistry, or pathology; therefore, courses in humanistic medicine have appeared to be more exhortative than substantive.

For a long time, much teaching about "the whole man" or even "social medicine" seemed to consist of normative prescriptions for tender loving care. It was operationally almost useless — that is, it did little for the student faced with the pragmatic problem of a particular patient with a particular set of symptoms — and, lacking data, it was inconsistent with the general scientific/technological milieu of the teaching hospital.[11]‡

Dysfunctional ideologies in medical schools promote the de-emphasis of primary care and holistic approaches. But the softness of the relevant data gives curriculum committees a rational basis for discrimination against courses in social medicine and comprehensive care. And the quality of the science is a dimension of technology.

When the work of human providers is replaced by machines, they may literally come between patients and staff, increasing physical and social distance. Communication devices in hospitals may make it unnecessary for nurses to respond to patients in person, and electronic history takers may displace live interviewers.[42] Such instruments can reduce the drudgery of work and expand human freedom, but they can also decrease face-to-face contact. The absence of human providers from the proximate space of patients may be alienating if it is interpreted as a cold impersonal affront to the patient's dignity.

Similarly, technology can affect the perceptions of health professionals. In intensive care, coronary care, and neonatal units, it may be questionable where the patient leaves off and some mechanical apparatus begins. Since many of these patients are comatose, heavily sedated, asleep, or irrational, they may more easily be perceived as extensions of tubes, respirators, and signaling devices than as human beings.[19]

Some might argue that the ICU dehumanizes the staff by depersonalizing services and inflating the relative importance of machinery. But patient needs and demands in these units can be so intense[1] that the presence of hardware at the interface can protect health workers from incessant emotional erosion. Yet, professionals and patients can become too dependent on hard technology. The fact that it exists within their purview combined with the monetary investment it represents provide strong incentives to use *it* instead of person tools.

In assessing the dehumanizing potential of technology, it is important to recognize how the computer can threaten the privacy of patients and providers.[7] The readiness and comprehensiveness of pooled data can tempt various people who have access to monitor the health status or behavior of particular individuals, for illegitimate as well as legitimate purposes.

If medical technologies are humanizing because they prolong life and reduce pain, the widespread prevalence of iatrogenic injury[32] from their use

---

‡Our quotation was taken from an earlier draft of Geiger's paper.

is a form of dehumanization. Iatrogenic illnesses are partly the fault of the social order and forces within — the profit priorities of drug and equipment manufacturers, the teaching and research priorities of academic institutions, the break-even incentives of non-profit hospitals, the "make-a-living" motivations of surgeons, radiologists, chemotherapists, and other technicians, and the "cure me" demands of patients. These vested interests promote the overuse and misuse of technologies. But the problem also stems from imperfections in the medical art.

Such imperfections are not necessarily distributed equally among well-to-do and indigent patients. The greater resources of the elite can lead to over-consultation, over-doctoring, over-medication, and over-surgery.[23] But poorer patients may lack the time and means to participate in long and involved therapeutic encounters in which the value of different regimens can be properly assessed.

4. *Self-Fulfilling Prophecies.*   The belief that technology per se carries the seeds of dehumanization can be a self-fulfilling expectation. Policy makers and managers of care may assume without question that dehumanization is an unavoidable by-product of technological advance — a trade off or sacrifice to be accepted as inevitable. Negation of this prophecy becomes impossible if there is no quest for benign or humanizing alternatives.

Medical tools may have a power of their own, but the use of that power is controlled by people. Beliefs which attribute superhuman capabilities to machines and medications tend to absolve caretakers and careseekers of responsibility for their actions. This process of abdication is itself dehumanizing, and it allows other dehumanizing consequences of technology to go unopposed because those who could resist are psychologically impotent.

Another self-fulfilling belief is the idea that effective and efficient utilization of technology necessitates aggregation of equipment and expertise. As more and more health professionals accept this belief, they merge themselves and their tools into centralized clusters, leaving the urban and rural hinterlands unattended or attended by those outside the in-group.[17,32] The expected style of practice for highly trained professionals may become the only style as they seek the geographic company of colleagues they respect. It then becomes impossible to test the effectiveness of alternative approaches, and aggregation becomes its own justification. As we point out below, centralization per se need not be dehumanizing. But the pressure on providers to congregate means that they are not really free to choose a solo-isolated mode of practice, and the options of patients are constricted as well.

Recommendations.   Strategies for change stem naturally from the foregoing discussion. If the dehumanizing effects of technology are to be reduced and counterbalanced, policy makers must challenge vested interests and attempt to alter attitudes and actions of the public at large and those who make their living from medical care and its tools. We offer the following guidelines:

1. The primary justification for the use of a medical technology should be its contribution to the well-being of *patients*.
2. In setting investment priorities, policy makers should compare the potential contributions of various medical technologies and nontechnological approaches. If "clean living"§ adds more productive years to human lives than transplants, dialysis, and heart surgery, techniques to encourage "clean living" should be given higher priority than after-the-fact heroics.
3. Added increments of life should be appraised in terms of their quality, not simply in terms of their quantity.
4. The potential harm of applying a medical technology must be incorporated into assessments of relative value.
5. Technologies which appreciably enhance the well-being of patients should be made universally available to those in need, within the limits imposed by distributive justice. If resources are scarce, policy makers must balance the health needs of special groups against those of society as a whole, allocating resources accordingly. Distributive justice may be accomplished through categorical aid or through some type of national health insurance which would subsidize necessary diagnostic work-ups, therapy, and medication (*e.g.*, antihypertensive drugs, polio vaccines, insulin).
6. Consumers of care should be encouraged to increase their understanding of health, illness, appropriate therapies, and the management 'of care. Information should be supplied by health professionals and by sources independent of the health-care establishment.[23] Extending the knowledge and skills of consumers should deflate the mystique of the medical professions and heighten their accountability.
7. The option of patients to use or refuse particular technologies should be made meaningful by insuring fully informed consent without coercion. Formal procedures to obtain consent should be deritualized and divorced as far as possible from pressures and persuasions of the therapeutic context. Where necessary, ombudsmen should be called upon to buttress the power of patients vis à vis practitioners and researchers with a stake in therapy.

Refusing to prolong a life of pain without hope should also be the patient's perogative. But the irrevocability of death makes it absolutely imperative that decisions to terminate life be made voluntarily and that they be protected from the intrusion of economic considerations.
8. The computer's threat to the privacy of patients and providers calls for foolproof safeguards. There must be meaningful restrictions on the type of information stored on computers and its availability. Access should be a privilege (not a right) dependent on the informed consent of the vulnerable parties.
9. Where modern science and specialization result in fragmentation of care,

---

§The term "clean living" is a synonym for certain habits that result in longer life — moderate drinking, no smoking, regular mealtimes, eight hours of sleep a night, etc.[6]

allocation of resources to primary and integrating forms of care should help neutralize the negative effects of fragmentation.

10. Technologies should be appraised on their merits, not in terms of their prestige. If person-to-person approaches are at least as effective as harder therapies and no more costly, their use should be encouraged.

To improve the quality of the "softer" technologies, resources should be channeled into research and development. The components of tender loving care deserve to be identified, evaluated, fashioned into more effective tools, and made a more legitimate part of the armamentarium of health professionals. If the utility of comprehensive care (holistic therapy) is empirically validated, forging its passage into professional schools is likely to become easier.[11]

11. Technologies which alleviate the drudgery of health care should be promoted, but any dehumanizing consequences of substituting hardware for people must be considered and countered. The flavor of human beings can be re-introduced in a different form if patients miss the presence of people. Lay persons might creatively fill the gap reducing the chance of tasks becoming routinized through professional performance.[9,23]

12. The technological dehumanization of providers needs special attention. If the prestige and sense of importance from working in an ICU do not compensate for the psychological erosion that occurs there, other means of compensatory humanization must be sought. The answer may lie in shorter hours, more reliefs, greater participation in decision making, greater contact with colleagues, or other solutions.

The best approach to humanizing care is to structure reward systems so that humanizing behaviors have visible payoffs and dehumanizing behaviors visible costs.‖ Thus, Rashi Fein proposes that under national health insurance, bonuses might be offered HMOs as incentives for effective preventive care.[23]¶

Humanization of care seldom suffices as its own reward, and exhortation is essentially useless unless it fronts for power.[23] At the symposium, participants debated the relative effectiveness of change agents from inside and outside medical institutions. Jack Geiger distrusted insiders, but Price Cobbs feared that reliance on outsiders is a cop-out that further victimizes victims.[9,10] The group finally concluded that to humanize care, health professionals and consumers must join forces in alliances of power.

Implications of Centralization

A popular explanation for dehumanization in health care (and for dehumanization in almost every sphere of modern life**) has to do with *scale*.

‖e.g., Loss of research funds if protocols are not approved by human subjects committees.
¶e.g., If 90 per cent of pregnant patients associated with the HMO received prenatal care by the third month, the group would get a financial bonus from the government.
**Such as education, welfare services, retail merchandising, law enforcement, penology, and with the advent of computer dating, even courtship.

Thus, Roslyn Lindheim observes: "If we talk about the need to personalize care and then design medical centers that are so large and impersonal they defy human scale, we are operating under a different set of priorities from those we profess."[32]

The problem of scale may derive from a purely economic and instrumental approach to human affairs whereby ostensibly "too few" are responsible for servicing ostensibly "too many." On the other hand, there may be an abundance of providers, but the bigness of the enterprise can give the impression that no one is personally interested in patients.

BIGNESS AND BUREAUCRACY

The preferred means for dispensing services in large-scale organizations is that of bureaucracy — a legal-administrative specification and implementation of clearly differentiated rules, procedures, and priorities so that service can be rendered in accord with *universalistic* rather than *particularistic* criteria.[35]‡‡ From the standpoint of justice through equality, universalism is humanizing, but it stresses the replaceability of human beings, not their unique attributes.[19]

Even where the bureaucratic ideal of equality of service in a context of optimal efficiency is achieved, the conviction persists that the sheer size of the enterprise will inevitably lead to dehumanization and related interpersonal pathologies. Indeed, some analysts maintain, not altogether without reason, that the more perfect the attainment of the bureaucratic ideal the greater the likelihood of a dehumanized service, as if to suggest that a certain amount of "getting around the rules" by clients and "looking the other way" by staff are necessary if a decent human standard in the giving of the service is to survive.[24]

Whether the bureaucratic solution to the problem of scale succeeds or fails in terms of its own logic, the belief is deeply entrenched that bigness and bureaucracy inevitably convert person-to-person relationships into relationships between objects, with all that this entails (e.g., manipulation, insensitivity, condescension, and perhaps plastic sociability). Hence, the popularity of recommendations to decentralize services, or decrease the number of clients, or possibly to diminish their need (through preventive care).

Such arguments are obviously oversimplified. There is good reason to believe that largeness of scale is neither a necessary or sufficient condition for dehumanized care. Other influences appear to play an important role. These include the dehumanizing effects of technology discussed above and such factors as the following:
1. Discontinuities in care stemming from high turnover and shifting about of practitioners and patients; or from institutional priorities which interfere

---

‡‡*i.e.*, Criteria that are applicable to all people in the relevant category, not to particular individuals as such.

with repeated consultations between the same providers and patients, and with the dovetailing of expectations this fosters.

2. Pronounced social class differences between practitioners and clients — differences in thought, language, and life styles — which give rise to problems of communication, interaction, and empathy. Such problems frequently occur when upper-middle-class physicians treat working-class patients or when lower-class aides in nursing homes offend the sensibilities of patients who were once well-to-do.

3. Standardized approaches which overlook unique characteristics that form the essence of individualized treatment.

4. Administrative arrangements which mask the visibility of staff actions and make subsequent accountability problematic.

5. Client passivity and feelings of powerlessness which may reflect subjective awe or exclusion from decision-making processes regarding care.

6. Physical designs of health-care settings (e.g., bench-lined, bile-green corridors devoid of decoration or recreational detractions) which can generate or aggravate a sense of depersonalization.

7. Staff attitudes, outlook, and morale that can undermine compassionate care or overcome obstacles to delivering it.

Several of these influences such as discontinuities in care, uniform approaches, invisibility of staff actions, and client passivity are probably exacerbated by bigness and bureaucracy. This means that patients and providers in large-scale delivery systems have to be especially alert and resistant to pressures toward dehumanization.

The interpersonal problems associated with scale will undoubtedly plague the HMOs blueprinted for the future. Clyde Pope's research in a prepaid group practice sheds light on the satisfaction and dissatisfaction of patients in one type of HMO setting.

THE KAISER-PERMANENTE EXPERIENCE

As Greenlick points out, a number of social planners have accepted prepaid group practice as the best approach to organizing America's health care.[15] The government's development of the "health maintenance organization" or HMO concept as part of its national health program gave official support to the prepaid group practice model.

When a medical care system, rather than an individual practitioner, assumes responsibility for the care of the patient, the relationship between provider and patient becomes less intimate. Such relationships give practitioners greater protection from exploitation than primary ones do. Within an organized system the individual provider does not need to be available at the beck and call of the patient nor does he or she need to be greatly concerned about the consequences of rejecting an inappropriate demand from a patient.

Similarly, in an organized system, a patient need not feel personally beholden to a physician because of an important service rendered or because a medical need interrupts the physician's family life. Nor do patients need to feel disloyal if someone other than their regular physician cares for them or if they choose to obtain a second opinion or to change doctors altogether. Furthermore, patients can legitimately feel that it is the system's responsibility to meet their medical care needs and that they have a right to service.

When an organization is the provider, patients as members may individually or collectively prevail upon its administration so as to increase their own satisfaction with services. The nature of organized relationships makes it easier for people to confront each other as "role occupants" rather than as personalities. Of course, this also increases the potential for depersonalization or dehumanization.

The Kaiser-Permanente program, the largest and probably best known of the prepaid group practices, is the prototype of the HMO. For several years the Oregon region of this program has been the focus of social and economic research by a number of investigators. Clyde Pope has been using a survey approach to evaluate the Kaiser program from the perspective of current and former members.

Reporting on their experience with the system, members and former members appear relatively satisfied with the quality of care, the facilities, the characteristics or behavior of physicians and other personnel, and, except for the scheduling of appointments, with general access to care. The greatest majority of former members terminated their membership because they moved out of the area or changed jobs wherein their insurance options did not include Kaiser.

Because the system offers the services of approximately 200 physicians and well over 1,000 other personnel to nearly 200,000 members, the potential for depersonalization is high. The two ongoing surveys, therefore, are designed to obtain information pertinent to this issue.

Although the respondents express general satisfaction with the program, they also have a number of specific criticisms. However, their comments suggest that depersonalization and dehumanization are not inevitable consequences of large-scale delivery systems. Only a little more than ten per cent of current members offer complaints that could be considered criticisms of impersonality. A somewhat greater proportion of former members have such complaints, but very few say they terminated for that reason. Other criticisms are far more numerous. The most frequent concerns appointment lag — that too much time elapses from the day one schedules an appointment until one actually sees a physician. Waiting time in the clinics is the second most common complaint, though far less frequent than the first.

The operating rules or procedures established by the organization are also criticized: the rotation or reassignment of physicians among clinics, the use of a message center for getting in touch with specific physicians, and the policy of informing patients of laboratory and x-ray results only when findings are positive. None of these items by itself is mentioned by many members, but collectively they account for a large proportion of the complaints.‡‡

Of course, as with all systems, people do learn how to manipulate or otherwise get around some of these rules or standard operating procedures. When asked what they do or would do if they could not get an appointment soon enough, respondents commonly say: "walk-in without an appointment." And available evidence indicates this is exactly what patients do. Additionally, patients report that they overstate or inaccurately state a problem to the appointment clerk, or imply an emergency, or go to the emergency clinic after hours, or call their regular physician directly, bypassing the appointment and message centers. Even though most respondents do not think the organization expects it, the majority of members indicate that they have a physician they consider their own, or their children's, regular doctor.

For the members of Kaiser-Permanente, the most important health-care goal is to have ensured access to care at the least possible cost.[15] The general satisfaction of the Portland members probably reflects the realization of this goal. Difficulties in scheduling appointments and long waits in doctor's offices are not new experiences to most people. But guaranteed care at familiar locations on a 24-hour basis, seven days a week, with low and predictable out-of-pocket costs, *is* something new to many people. These advantages may compensate for problems that might otherwise evoke more dissatisfaction with the system. It should also be noted that the Portland region may or may not be typical of the six highly autonomous regions of this prepaid plan. However, the Portland region certainly qualifies as a large-scale delivery system.

The Kaiser-Permanente organization recognizes that depersonalization and dehumanization are problems that can threaten the success of the program. And like all organizations, this group is committed to its own survival. But it is difficult if not impossible for an institution to *decree* the level of personal warmth necessary to humanize relationships. Structural alternatives must be devised. For example, Kaiser-Permanente has developed a program for monitoring membership satisifaction and responding to the problems identified. It has increased the activities and status of the membership relations department; it has disseminated information within the organization regarding membership satisfaction; and it has established a program to increase the involvement of personnel in meeting organizational objectives.

---

‡‡Jan Howard believes that complaints about waiting time, rotation of physicians, and message centers might well be considered criticisms of depersonalization even though the term or a synonym is not used. In rebuttal, Clyde Pope argues that these particular procedures are criticized infrequently and that when an issue like physician rotation is mentioned in open-ended comments, the context of the statement suggests that depersonalization is not the factor being criticized. There is no suggestion that the event is demeaning or a threat to the patient's integrity. The basic concern is patient inconvenience or a similiar issue. Thirdly, respondents tend to criticize specific incidents rather than general characteristics of the system.

Recommendations. While depersonalization is only one issue, it is significant because it relates so strongly to the issue of psychosocial effectiveness which is a vital component of overall organizational effectiveness. We, therefore, recommend that HMOs like Kaiser-Permanente try to structure their organizations to take account of depersonalization and its various manifestations and to respond to patient needs for humanism. We also suggest that such procedures as rotation of physicians, nonreporting of negative findings, and pooling of messages be re-evaluated periodically. Where possible, continuity of care and comprehensive communication should take precedence over efficiency and economy.

Implications of Self-Help Care

Many people believe that humanization of care requires greater participation of patients in the care process. It is, therefore, important to understand the self-help movement because its objective is to take certain aspects of physical and mental care out of the control of professionals and make them the legitimate domain of persons involved in the receipt of services. Instead of relying on professionals to define the nature of health problems, prescribe regimens and offer therapy, lay participants in self-help organizations assume these responsibilities for themselves. They firmly believe that persons who experience and share certain health problems have the capacity to manage them more effectively than professional experts.

Self-help groups are organized by laypersons around specific problems. A variety of groups exist to assist persons afflicted by particular illnesses (e.g., Emphysema Anonymous, Committee to Combat Huntington's Disease, mastectomy recovery organizations). Others provide routine or preventive obstetric and gynecologic care and education (e.g., International Childbirth Education Association, home birth centers, La Leche League, self-help gynecology clinics). Numerous peer self-help organizations seek to improve mental health and to overcome problems viewed as psychological (e.g., Alcoholics Anonymous, Recovery, Inc., Emotional Health Anonymous, Associated Rational Thinkers, Synanon, Overeaters Anonymous, Parents Anonymous, feminist therapy groups).[3,25,30,37,38]

WHY SELF-HELP?

Self-help care has emerged to fill serious gaps in service and to offer alternatives to forms of traditional care which are viewed as ineffective, inappropriate, or too expensive. Initially, most organizations grew out of the efforts of a few individuals who had suffered personally from poor care. Many of these neglected or inappropriately treated problems involve stigmatized conditions such as alcoholism, drug addiction, obesity, and mental illness. Others involve social adjustment to chronic conditions (heart disease, arthritis) that falls between the cracks in technocratized western medicine.

Despite many differences in organizational structure, political ideology, political activism, and characteristics of participants, these groups share key features which have important implications for understanding needed changes in traditional health care. By examining these features we may begin to develop ideas for restructuring certain parts of the larger health care system.

KEY FEATURES OF SELF-HELP

1. *Lay Control.*   In contrast to most health care, all aspects of self-help groups are controlled by laypersons who share a common problem or condition. Professionals are not sought out for leadership roles or provision of services. In fact, self-help represents an attack on professionalism which is perceived as elitist and too distant from the realities of daily life. Professionals are often excluded for fear they may attempt to dominate and wrest authority and control from laypersons.

2. *Experiential Base of Expertise.*   In traditional health-care settings professionals seldom suffer from the conditions they treat. Self-helpers believe that only persons who share the common experience are qualified to offer assistance. Individuals cannot be experts on the basis of professional training alone because professionals often fail to understand the patient's total situation unless they have personally experienced the same condition. Accounts of professional ignorance and insensitivity are important aspects of self-help folklore.

Because of the experiential base of expertise, all participants are considered potentially able to give as well as receive help, in keeping with the shared values and perspectives of the group. The only professionals who are allowed to participate are those who are bona fide members or who show full acceptance of the self-help perspective.

3. *Criticism of Traditional Theories and Practices.*   Self-helpers often challenge traditional medical theories and practices. For example, mental health groups generally reject Freudian theories of emotional disturbance and focus on pragmatic therapy based on underlying principles of learning theory.[25] Feminist self-help groups challenge traditional psychological theories about women and reject the traditional boundaries of medical practice.[38] Other organizations such as the Committee to Combat Huntington's Disease have undermined false assumptions about the effects of certain illnesses (e.g., that a particular condition leads to mental incompetence), and they have encouraged more accurate diagnosis.[16]

4. *Demystification.*   Self-help groups demystify health care by presenting problems in understandable everyday language. Some publish their own educational material and strive to increase the ability of participants to utilize health care systems effectively and appropriately when necessary.[2] In addition, the ideology that each participant is potentially a provider of care reduces the idealization of health professionals.

5. *Personal Involvement and Sharing.*   The core of self-help programs is the sharing of personal concerns. Professional distance, neutrality, and privacy

are replaced by open revelation of problems in a group setting. The atmosphere is supportive but not necessarily nonjudgmental; for self-help groups often develop strong moral stands and prohibitions against behavior that is regarded as deviant, self-destructive, or irresponsible. Expressions of moral judgment are therefore viewed as expressions of concern for the well-being of individuals. Although groups organize around specific problems, participants are encouraged to share their general problems in living. Thus, physical, emotional, and social adjustment are considered on an ongoing basis.

6. *Support Systems.*   Self-help groups offer individuals the opportunity to develop support systems and mutual-aid networks unavailable in traditional medical settings which are typically structured to maintain the privacy of patients. Self-helpers develop social ties with others, sharing similar problems or conditions, and call upon each other in times of need. In many respects such groups serve the function of an extended family.

7. *Costs.*   Administrative costs are minimized by utilizing volunteer labor. Paid staff members (recruited from the ranks of participants) usually receive low salaries. To cover operating expenses, self-help groups rely largely on donations or payment-in-service in lieu of fees. Additional funds come from foundations and government grants.§§ If set fees are suggested or required, they are typically nominal and can be waived in cases of hardship. Thus, potential recruits are rarely barred from participation because of poverty.

IMPLICATIONS OF SELF-HELP FOR HUMANIZING HEALTH CARE

The concept of self-help points to certain inadequacies in traditional approaches to care. These deficiencies stem from the fact that professionals exclusively control research and treatment of many health problems. To humanize health care, persons who have first-hand experience with particular diseases or conditions should be involved in defining areas of needed research and evaluating the adequacy of theories and clinical practices. In addition, laypersons are a tremendous resource for providing health care.

Self-help groups underscore the need for holistic approaches to health. Regardless of the specific problem or condition for which individuals seek help, they experience their states of being physically, emotionally, and socially. To separate out these components and send patients to specialists who treat only one aspect of a condition fragments the individual and dehumanizes the entire health restoring process, making it less effective. From the patient's perspective, the personal element can be as important or even more important than the technological facets of treatment.

Finally, the self-help movement questions the necessity for highly-paid professionals where persons with less training seem to have equal success.[25]

---

§§Some groups accept government grants; others are wary of outside control.[3]

And making health care available at low cost extends access to persons who cannot afford private professional care.

Recommendations.   How might the self-help approach be used to improve and humanize certain aspects of the health care system? Broad general recommendations are difficult to make, for self-help groups vary both in effectiveness and propensity to work collaboratively with professionals. Some self-help gynecology groups welcome professionals; others accept only those who are women; and some exclude all professionals qua professionals. In contrast, most organizations focusing on specific diseases work closely with professionals. Even self-help groups at the radical extreme are receptive to developing alliances with traditional providers of care if these providers show respect for the group and assure its autonomy.

Recognizing that our recommendations are more relevant to some groups than others, we suggest the following:

1. Additional research on contemporary self-help programs would elucidate the range of problems which have been treated successfully and unsuccessfully; the effectiveness of various therapeutic approaches; the consequences of size, structure, and political activism; and the categories of persons receptive to lay-group care.

2. Laypersons involved in effective self-help groups might be recruited to teach in professional training programs and to supervise students in self-help field placements. (This has been done successfully with gynecology groups and drug treatment programs.)

3. Health planners and legislators might consider revising licensing laws and insurance practices which determine what categories of personnel can provide care and who can be reimbursed by public or private insurance. Serious thought should be given to minimizing distinctions between medical and non-medical personnel offering similar and equally effective services.

4. New working relationships between professionals, paraprofessionals, and laypersons who offer services in specialized areas need to be developed. Perhaps some synthesis of successful self-help working relationships could be used to improve upon the currently popular models of "maximum feasible participation," "therapeutic community," and "separate spheres of authority."

5. Through health education programs and the mass media, laypersons should be encouraged to take more active roles in health care. Simultaneously, physicians might be encouraged to increase patient involvement in the decision-making process and to work more closely with patients in laying out and monitoring treatment strategies. The experiences of self-help groups could be instructive in this regard.

FOOTNOTES

1. Benoliel, J.Q.: "The realities of work: Commentary on Howard
   Leventhal's information-processing model," *In* Humanizing Health Care.
   Howard J., and Strauss, A., Eds. New York, John Wiley and Sons, 1975.

2. Berkeley Women's Health Collective: Feeding ourselves. Boston, New England Free Press, 1972. See also, The Boston Women's Health Book Collective: Our Bodies, Ourselves — a Book by and for Women. New York: Simon and Schuster, 1973; Lang, R. *The Birth Book*. Ben Lomond, California: Genesis Press, 1972; Alcoholics Anonymous World Services, Inc.: Twelve steps and twelve traditions. New York, AA World Service, Inc., 1965.

3. Borman, L.D., Ed.: Explorations in Self-Help and Mutual Aid. Evanston, Ill., Center for Urban Affairs, Northwestern University, 1975.

4. Bullough, B.: Poverty, ethnic identity and preventive health care. J. Health Soc. Behav. 13: 347, 1972.

5. Carlson, R.J.: The end of machine. New York, John Wiley and Sons, 1975.

6. "Clean Living — Long Life." *San Francisco Chronicle*, September 22, 1975.

7. Department of Health, Education, and Welfare. Records, Computers, and the Rights of Citizens. Report of the Secretary's Advisory Committee on Automated Personal Data Systems, DHEW Publication No. (OS) 73-94, Washington, D.C., U.S. Printing Office, 1973; Springarn, N.D.: Confidentiality. Report of the Conference on Confidentiality of Health Records, Key Biscayne, Florida, November 6-9, 1974. Washington, D.C., American Psychiatric Association, 1975.

8. Fein, R.: *In* Howard J., and Tyler, C.C.: Comments on dehumanization: Caveats, dilemmas, and remedies. *In* Howard J., and Strauss, A., Eds., *op. cit.*

9. Freidson, E.: Increasing choice within limits: Commentary on Donald Kennedy's model for change. *In* Howard, J., and Strauss, A., Eds. *op. cit.*

10. _____: Profession of medicine, a study of the sociology of applied knowledge. New York, Dodd, Mead, and Company, 1970: Davis, F.: Uncertainty in medical prognosis, clinical and functional. *In* Scott, W.R., and Volkart, E.H., Eds. *Medical Care: Readings in the Sociology of Medical Institutions*. New York, John Wiley and Sons, 1966.

11. Geiger, H.J.: The causes of dehumanization in health care and prospects for humanization. *In* Howard J., and Strauss, A., Eds., *op. cit.*

12. Gerson, E.M.: On "quality of life." University of California at San Francisco, March, 1975 (unpublished working paper).

13. Goffman, E.: Asylums. New York, Anchor, 1961.

14. Gray, B.H.: Human Subjects in Medical Experimentation. New York, John Wiley and Sons, 1975.

15. Greenlick, M.R.: The impact of prepaid group practice on American medical care: A critical evaluation. Ann. Am. Acad. Polit. Soc. Sci. 399:100, 1972. Other references that served as a basis for ideas in this section include: Donabedian, A.: An evaluation of prepaid group practice. Inquiry 6:3, 1969. Etzioni, A., Ed.: *Complex Organizations: A Sociological Reader*. New York, Holt, Rinehart and Winston, 1961; Katz, D., and Kahn, R.L.: *The Social Psychology of Organizations*. New York, John Wiley & Sons, 1966; Weinerman, E.R.: Patient's perceptions of group medical care: A review and analysis of studies on choice and utilization of prepaid group practice plans. Am. J. Public Health 54:880, 1964.

16. Guthrie, M.: *In* Borman, L.D., Ed., *op. cit.*

17. Hall, O.: The informal organization of the medical profession. Can. J. Econ. Politic. Sci. 12:30, 1946.

18. Howard, J.: Humanization and dehumanization of health care. *In* Reich, W.T., Ed.: Encyclopedia of Bioethics. Washington, D.C., Georgetown University, forthcoming.
19. _____: Humanization and dehumanization of health care: A conceptual view. *In* Howard, J., and Strauss, A., Eds., *op. cit.*
20. _____: Race differences in hypertension mortality trends: Differential drug exposure as a theory. Milbank Mem. Fund Q. 43:202, 1965.
21. _____: A sociologist's perspective on ethical issues in health care management. *In* Proceedings of the Seventeenth Annual Symposium on Hospital Affairs. Chicago, University of Chicago Press, 1976.
22. _____, and Strauss, A., Eds.: Humanizing Health Care. New York, John Wiley and Sons, 1975.
23. _____, and Tyler, C.C.: Comments on dehumanization: caveats, dilemmas, and remedies. *In* Howard J., and Strauss, A., Eds., *Ibid.*
24. Hughes, E.: Men and Their Work. Glencoe, Ill., The Free Press, 1958.
25. Hurvitz, N.: "Peer self-help psychotherapy groups. *In* The Sociology of Psychotherapy, Roman, P., and Trice, H.M. Eds. New York, Jason Aronson, 1974.
26. Jonsen, A.R.: Sounding board: Scientific medicine and therapeutic choice. N. Engl. J. Med. 292:126, 1975.
27. Kennedy, D.A.: Adaptation to more humanizing forms of health care. *In* Howard J., and Strauss, A., Eds., *op. cit.*; Crichton, M.: Five Patients. New York, Bantom, 1970.
28. Lee, P.R.: *In* Howard, J., and Tyler, C.C., *op. cit.*
29. Leventhal, H.: The consequences of depersonalization during illness and treatment: An information-processing model. *In* Howard J., and Strauss, A., Eds., *op. cit.*
30. Levin, L.S.: Self-Care in health, selected annotated bibliography. Unpublished paper, Department of Epidemiology and Public Health, Yale University, 1975.
31. Lewis, C.E.: A physician's perspective. *In* Howard J., and Strauss, A., Eds., *op. cit.*
32. Lindheim, R.: An architect's perspective. *In* Howard J., and Strauss, A., Eds., *op. cit.*
33. Mannes, M.: Last Rights: A Case for the Good Death. New York, William Morrow, 1974.
34. Mechanic, D.: Introduction. *In* Howard J., and Strauss, A., Eds., *op. cit.*
35. Parsons, T.: The Social System. New York, The Free Press, 1964; Illness and the role of the physician: A sociological perspective. *In* Personality in Nature, Society, and Culture. Kluckholn, C., and Murray, H.A., Eds. New York, Knopf, 1956.
36. Redlich, F.: *In* Howard, J., and Tyler, C.C., *op. cit.*
37. Ruzek S.K.: Emergent modes of utilization: Gynecological self-help. *In* Proceedings of the Conference Women and Their Health: Research Implications for a New Era. Olesen, V., Ed. In press.
38. _____: Women and health care: A bibliography with selected annotation. Evanston, Ill., The Program on Women, Northwestern University, Occasional Papers No. 1, 1975; The Feminist Counseling Collective: Feminist psychotherapy: A new method for fighting the social control of women. Am. J. Orthopsychiatry 44:187, 1974.

39. _____: The Women's health movement: Finding alternatives to traditional medical professionalism. Ph.D. dissertation, University of California at Davis, 1976.
40. Sanford, N., and Comstock, C., Eds.: Sanctions for Evil. San Francisco, Jossey-Bass, 1971.
41. Silverman, M., and Lee, P.R.: Pills, Profits, and Politics. Berkeley, University of California Press, 1974.
42. Slack, W. V., et al.: Patient-computer dialogue. N. Engl. J. Med. 286:1304, 1972.
43. Thomas, L.: Commentary: The future impact of science and technology on medicine. Bioscience 4:99, 1974.
44. Vail, D.: Dehumanization and the Institutional Career. Springfield, Ill., Charles C. Thomas, 1966.

The Implications of "Failure of Communication" in Hospitals

by E. Michael Bluestone

The time has come for us to admit to ourselves that the modern hospital has fallen on evil days. It has not, within living memory, been burdened so heavily with problems of all kinds which press in upon it and threaten its very humane ideology. Many of these problems are thrust upon us by external forces which are almost beyond our control. Others, however, originate on the premises and should be easier to resolve. Outstanding among the latter, if only because of its epidemology, is the one that is created by "failure of communication" which, in earlier years, went by the name of "human relations" as between the sick and those who serve them. This failure, by whatever name, becomes progressively more hurtful to the patient as the hospital expands, becomes more complex in its organisation, and is diverted from its essential purpose. Reluctance to deal with it face-to-face is a self-defeating reaction, particularly when it may be imposed by budgetary restraints in a time of austerity and retrenchment. Since a sovereign remedy for this institutional malady, and one that we have hesitated too long to use, is at hand, let us see why and how we should apply it.

The mere mention of communication-failure is embarrassing to many of us who feel that we can cope with it, and keep it within bounds, by conventional methods of organisation and administration. Some continue to believe that, like sin, it will always be with us in spite of anything we might do to counteract it. However, turning away from it can only end by tarnishing the image of the hospital which we prize so highly. Quite literally, we can talk ourselves out of it with the help of an administrative device, if it is properly adjusted to the normal limitations of human nature.

Communication-failure cannot be condoned in the presence of a variety of irritants which the hospital unwittingly generates in the course of its multiplying services. In one way or another, this failure aggravates the mental or physical condition of the patient — after he was admitted in the hope that, by words as well as by deeds, he would be sheltered from all harm, a hope which admits of no mental reservations on the part of the hospital.

The hospital — and this includes its allied institutions — is a product of its environment and subject to its influence, social, economic, and even political, for better or for worse. Moreover, the mechanical, biological and social sciences make their contributions to the advancement of the hospital in an escalating flow. But all of these increase the complexity of the

From *World Hospitals*, Vol. XIII, No. 3, 1977. By permission of the author and publisher.

institutional organisation and create problems, of which the one that goes by the name of "communication" becomes intensified and more demanding. The conscience of the hospital is involved here and it can be tested by its willingness and its ability to respond acceptably.

Communication, as a way of hospital life, is all the more compelling when you reflect that there is no surrounding activity of whatever nature which does not, in one way or another, come in contact with, influence — and benefit from — hospital service. Every profession, trade and occupation is called upon, sooner or later, to make its contribution to the hospital effort. In many useful ways, commerce and industry add their "know-how," and more, to hospital management. Within the hospital the efficiency-expert elaborates a graphic scheme of organisation which shows lines of authority and responsibility in stratified layers but, like "the letter of the law," it should be interpreted by "the spirit thereof." All departments and services overlap more or less — and in the interest of the patient who belongs on the diagram.

It takes more than prophetic vision in a rapidly changing world to build, equip and staff a hospital that will explain itself automatically to its clientele. Moreover, the certainty of obsolescence in all three of these categories is a reality to be reckoned with, if only because of its baneful influence on up-to-date medical care. Every hospital does indeed function under a number of built-in handicaps, animate and inanimate, which must be surmounted. These are facts which a sick person cannot be expected to understand without help from those who do. In any case, communication is far more productive in many ways than silence!

In circumstances like these the hospital cannot "muddle through" with impunity, either because of inertia, negativism, or myopia, in the expectation that grievances, voiced or unvoiced, will disappear if given a dose of "tincture of time." Experience has taught us that they may do so, but it has also taught us, with considerable embarrassment to us, that they usually do not. Rules and regulations multiply as a facile cure-all, but they must be applied selectively, in the patient's interest, and for no strictly disciplinary reason. In general, administrative legalisms must be softened by words which turn away wrath — words which have the soothing effect of an emollient, or of a lubricant which prevents friction. When unheeded or suppressed complaints promote fear and anxiety, there is no tranquilising drug which can compete with sympathetic communication in overcoming them. Peace of mind during hospitalised illness is all the more difficult for a sick person to attain because he is perforce a stranger among strangers in his temporary institutional abode, where the current hospital jargon is foreign to him.

The emotional shock of transfer from home to hospital needs, for its relief, the preventive use of communication. In its absence institutional effort, no matter how skilful otherwise, may be hampered, complicated and even nullified. Patients who leave the hospital prematurely, "against advice," are hurtful reminders of our neglect in this area of hospital management. It is a sobering thought that failure-of-communication never appears in an autopsy report — nor can you obtain permission to perform such an examination without putting your heart into the appeal!

The terminology used in hospitals, some of it with tongue-in-cheek or in the nature of an affectation, is at times reminiscent of the abstruse Latin in which prescriptions were written — in a bad hand — in an earlier generation. It covers a vocabulary which few patients can understand without a generous supply of synonyms by way of explanation. In general, the patient is in a "hospital" (a term which is becoming old-fashioned) even when he enters a "medical centre." Simple expressions like "semi-private" are difficult to defend, because privacy cannot be expressed in terms of a fraction. But we dare not forget that the patient is there only because he cannot be anywhere else under the demanding circumstances of his illness. He does not have a choice in the matter! And his spiritual co-operation must be actively sought.

Educational and research activity in the hospital which are, in effect, by-products of medical care, have a long list of precautions to observe about which the patient cannot be assumed to be knowledgeable without some persuasive form of communication. Nor can we expect his submissive co-operation where collective patient-service may be discriminative in the distribution of its bounty. Without inviting his understanding, how would you have him react to his competitive position? In all these situations there is a lesson to be learned from the do-it-yourself person who, in a different context, is misled into patronising the patient-medicine remedy, the virtues of which have been communicated to him in fulsome language by the popular "media." How much more would he, as a hospital patient, listen to more helpful advice when he is victimized by illness and ready to grasp at straws!

Relatives and friends have visiting privileges, read the newspapers and wait anxiously, hoping that the hospital will use its powers of salvation for their loved ones. They must therefore be included in the communication network when the chips are down, as they always are. Justice to everyone, like justice everywhere else, may not achieve perfection but it should at least be approximated by a healthy respect for emotion as well as logic. The fact that some patients are reluctant to look a gift-horse in the mouth when they are cast as supplicants — of fear reprisals — should influence our administrative relationships with them. Tradition is suggestive in hospitals but it is not mandatory. The hospital as well as the patient, is more secure when it shares legitimate information with him that will reinforce his efforts at orientation. It is wrong for us to lay the flattering unction to our souls that "the hospital knows best" and is entitled to unquestionable acceptance. What does it "know best"?

The higher one must go with a grievance in the hospital hierarchy (and the right to appeal is inalienable) the less time is available to deal definitively with it. The complaint may or may not be justifiable but the patient must be given the benefit of any doubt in dealing with it. Complaints from a variety of sources, depending on the ability of the administration to calm fears and anxieties, real or imagined, are inevitable in the nature of institutional service. One can temporise with such things, procrastinate, invoke the virtue of patience, or stand by the rule, but patients are patients! Unfortunately, the sick person — perhaps because of his illness, its character, duration, or prognosis — is either attractive to those who serve him and react accordingly, or he is not. Besides, repetitious routines tend to breed callosities. We anticipate conformity with the Hippocratic Oath, or the Prayer of Maimonides, from all graduating students of medicine, but similiar oaths and prayers of equal inspiration are not universally in evidence by which we can measure conformity in the hospital personnel. Nor can the patient forget, since he may be the victim of it, that the strike as an instrument of labour warfare may crush him between the proverbial millstones as it concentrates on the case for the staff as opposed to the case for the sick.

Official solicitation of critical comments, favourable or unfavourable after the discharge of the patient from the hospital, comes at the wrong time, in absentia, and it is therefore correspondingly diminished in value. A belated explanation, or apology, comes with poor grace, since the lapse cannot be rubbed out by wishful thinking postponed. Like the mother who quickly forgets her labour-pains after the birth of her baby, the patient is only too glad to be home again to have his grievances revived.

The subjection of the hospital to ill-informed criticism, public or private, which is so often more destructive than constructive, has become quite the fashion of late. It does however remind us of our failings and our vulnerability. It should be embarrassing, if not humiliating, to the management of institutions for the sick to find itself prodded by careless outsiders who view the hospital and all its works darkly, through the wrong side of their binoculars, superficially aware of the exigencies of hospital service. Newspaper criticism, which is at times quite helpful, is too often hasty, perversely newsworthy, out of balance, and technically difficult of refutation. It may well be generated by institutional silence which is misinterpreted at strategic moments. The readiness of the potential "consumer" to believe what he sees in print is explained by the old saw: "where there is smoke there is fire." And, "what goes down in print cannot be chopped out by an axe."

The diagnosis of "failure of communication" being established, what is the cure? The condition is too often chronic, which makes therapy all the more difficult. We now have an administrative device that should be easily refined for the special use of hospitals. Seldom used by the watch-dogs of political bureaucracies as more than a pious gesture, it should have a definitive test in our institutions for the sick. In proportion to its strong potential, it is relatively inexpensive, and the test should be made in a controlled setting, with the large hospital as the best social laboratory for the purpose.

There may indeed be an explanation for the delay in the formal incorporation of this device in those hospitals which have an efficient Social Service Department, a helpful chaplain, a board of dedicated trustees, a productive Public Relations Department, special-nurses (for those who can afford their services), and a socially-minded organisation generally, all of whom do the best they can with the limited time and energy at their disposal. Experience has, however, taught us that their capacity for extrusion beyond their borders and their terms-of-reference, is circumscribed in actual practice by the restrictive facts-of-life in the numerous cross-currents of the institution. The unifying function of communication as here outlined, where there may be cause for complaint, must be concentrated rather than diluted in the best interests of the sick.

There is much more to this elusive and challenging problem than meets the eye — and the other senses — as every conscientious hospital executive knows from his experience in his office and in the field. The solution of the human-relations problem here outlined is, faute de mieux, the establishment on the most generous terms of an autonomous, but overlapping, service which focuses sharply on each patient from beginning to end. Resort to this service may be solicited or unsolicited, and emanate from any source. If the hospital is fortunate enough to provide an extra-mural service (popularly known as Home Care) it should, of course, be included, though complaints from this source are far less than in the hospital proper, and for obvious reasons!

For the purpose of obtaining the maximum value of penetrating and understandable communication, an office should be located strategically for ready access. It should be in the hands of a mature and experienced functionary who is wise in hospital lore. His task will be the tactful normalisation of all communication affecting the care of the patient, and to keep it flowing. This cannot be accomplished by the customary expedients of pamphlets, formal standards of conduct and discipline which suggest inflexibility — all of them elaborated for the benefit of the "consumer" who enjoys the hospitality of a health "industry" which "delivers" service to him "COD."

This "floating" personality, whose further qualifications need not be itemised here, should be in a position where he can cross borders as required to effect his special purpose. He should have his ear to the ground, so to speak, in order to detect any irritant which might affect the patient's comfort and recovery adversely. His task should be to advocate, arbitrate, and help to adjust, all situations where loss of communication has occurred, or threatens to occur. His presence on the premises should supplement, and therefore ease, the work of all other services — and raise the guard of all of them as they converge on the patient's requirements. He will, in effect, be a go-between, a communication-factotum who is certainly no fifth wheel to the hospital wagon. He does, in fact, give stability to the four which they may lack.

The kind of personality that I have in mind is tentatively known by a name which may sound strange to the ears of the modern social engineer. If you can suggest a more descriptive name for him than "ombudsman" I shall be glad to hear it. But, whatever we call him, we need him on our staff because we are learning that, without him, we cannot discharge our obligations to our clients fully, or do full justice to the institutions that we represent.

I cannot close these remarks without repeating my reference to the multiplicity of serious problems which confront the hospitals of our time. Most of them, like the one here discussed, have long been with us, and they will continue to bedevil our paths until we come to grips with them boldly and imaginatively. By the dramatic change in our communication-system here recommended, the image of the hospital will reflect our efforts — and do much more than take the sting out of hospital criticism.

I have taught my students that you cannot save a drowning man from a distance — you must come close to him! We must come closer to our patients and know each of them by name as we still their apprehension — directly, if practicable, by deputy if not. The kind of sympathetic communication here recommended has for its goal the elimination of excessive distance wherever possible, including the kind of spiritual distance which so many sick people find intolerable. It is, in a way, the medical counterpart of the legal "amicus curiae." It is promisingly therapeutic — the kind that prevents scars — if only because it proves to the patient, and the public, that the hospital will leave no stone unturned in its effort to restore him to health and productivity at the earliest possible time.

Of Half Gods and Mortals: Aesculapian Authority

Beatrice J. Kalisch

O you that are half gods, lengthen that life . . . turn o'er all the volumes of your mysterious Aesculapian science.[1]

A recent and personal encounter with illness and hospitalization reminded me of the above line in Philip Massinger's play of 1622, *The Virgin-Martyer*. I can testify that Aesculapius, the god of medicine in ancient Roman mythology, is alive and well today and working in medical care delivery settings, U.S.A.

As I entered the hospital, I glanced with a practiced eye at the surroundings and judged that everything looked the same as it always did. But soon I found that the experience of being a patient was like suddenly being lowered to the bottom of a well or raised to the top of a tower; the view of the same places and the same people drastically changed. For me, the most revealing and surprising insights occurred as a direct result of the relationship between myself and the physician. These revelations derived from one important concern throughout my hospitalization; my loss of control and lack of power to determine the events that affected me.

Active-Passive Continuum

As any two people interact, each person assumes a degree of activity and passivity. To the extent that one person is overly active, the other individual must become passive, or a clash occurs. The activity-passivity dimension determines who will be in control, the passive partner giving way to the more active one. Control also determines the nature of the decision-making process between two people. Thus, in a patient-physician relationship, if the patient is totally passive and immobilized (as, for example, during surgery), the surgeon assumes all of the activity, and there is virtually no interaction. The patient is a passive object, wholly submissive to the activity of the physician — a state of affairs which is obviously essential. Even when the patient is conscious and capable of reasoning and feeling, the physician may still exercise full control; he issues orders, and the patient is expected to follow along submissively.

On the other end of the continuum, a patient may assume a highly active role in the interaction, and the physician a totally passive stance. It may be difficult to imagine such a circumstance, and many would

consider it altogether unprofessional. Yet it does happen, as Duff and
H̶o̶l̶l̶i̶n̶g̶s̶h̶e̶a̶d̶ have documented in their exhaustive study of hospitals,
nurses:

. . . . ̶t̶e̶d̶ to protect their position as physician to the patient,
but they were not always free to use their best medical judgment. Many
physicians responded to the demands of the sick persons or their families
even when such demands had little to do with solving the patient's problems;
such demands commonly involved hospitalization, a "dictated" diagnosis, and
inappropriate therapy. The physician feared loss of status and income as well as
involvement in the problems of the patients.[2]

In this last instance, the patient is controlling the physician. Thus, we see
there are two possible models of physician-patient relationships: one based
on what is known as "aesculapian authority," and the other based on joint
participation.

Aesculapian Model

Where along this continuum of activity-passivity do most patient-physician
relationships fall? In the vast majority of instances, the physician holds
practically all of the control. In fact, the power he wields is so remarkably
potent that it has been specifically labeled as "aesculapian authority" by
Paterson.[3,4] It is utilized to convince patients that they are indeed "sick" and,
furthermore, that they must submit to various treatments, hospitalization,
and curtailment of normal activities.

For the person who is ill, this authority is greater than any other existing
power — at least, within that particular context and for that particular
moment. And he responds by meekly following along with what is ordered,
no matter how embarrassing, dangerous, or painful it may be. People who
are ordinarily aggressive turn passive, the dominant become submissive,
and the boisterous yield to silence. Outrages are tolerated from physicians
that would not be acceptable for a second from anyone else. The most
surprising and perplexing characteristic of this power is that it is invisible;
most people are totally unaware that it exists.

According to Paterson, aesculapian authority combines three different
kinds of authority, which accounts for its extreme potency. First, the
physician carries the authority of an expert, as is true of all people who have
the knowledge and skills essential for rendering a needed service valued by
society. An auto mechanic, for example, possessess an expertise thought to
be essential by most people; he is looked upon as an important authority
figure, at least, within the specific context of having one's car repaired. As
contrasted with the advice of the physician, however, we find it relatively
easy to reject the auto mechanic's suggestions. Granted, the seriousness of
the medical enterprise accounts for a portion of this difference, but not all of
it by any means. The physician wields something more than authority by
expertise.

Part of this super power is morally based, derived from the Hippocratic
oath. It gives the physician the right to control the patient because he is

believed to be morally committed to act for the good of his patients. He is a professional, guided by certain ethical principles and thus believed to act in the client's interest rather than his own. The thought that he might not do his very best never occurs to most people.

Beyond this, there is a third type of power, perhaps of major significance here. The result of tradition that dates back to centuries ago when medicine was a product of "natural philosophy," this power stems from the concept that the physician has license to control by reason of God-given grace. People believe — in a vague and almost unconscious way — that he has special connections with the world of the unknown, philosophically and spiritually.

For the layman, in contrast, medicine is still mysterious and unpredictable, set apart from normal human affairs. The key element that sustains this attitude is the arbitrary nature of life and death. In other words, it is the patient's fear of death and his desire to live, along with the conviction that the physician has special powers withheld from ordinary mortals, that causes the average person to believe that the physician has more going for him than expertise alone. It is somewhat suggestive of the tribal medicine man, and actually the physician does assume a half-godlike role.

I am reminded of a meeting where one of the speakers asked the audience: "What do you think the initials M.D. really stand for?" After a few moments of suspenseful silence, he answered his own question: "Minor Deity, of course." No one failed to get the point, since the privileged status attributed to physicians (how often do they get a parking ticket?) and the high order of egotism which typifies their behavior immediately came to everyone's mind. But beyond this it is apparent that this priestly role is utilized as part of the "bedside manner" for the purpose of persuading the patient to do what is "best" as diagnosed by the physician.

Only One Choice

As a result, the health care system is set up so that the patient has only one major choice — that of primary care or first-line physician. And this choice, it might be said, is usually based on such unreliable information as a friend's recommendation: "He's a good doctor." Few individuals know such basic facts as where their physician earned his medical degree, his years of experience and in what settings, and whether or not he is board certified.

After this initial choice, most decisions are made for the patient by that physician. This includes the choice of treatment, as well as the choice of specialists for referral or no referrals at all. Even the choice of hospitals is often determined for the patient.

This is quite a departure from other instances of consumer behavior. When an individual wishes to buy a new car, for instance, he not only determines which dealership he wants to patronize but also what he really would like in the way of a car and how much he is willing to pay for it. These basic decisions are not made for him, even though salesmen may inspire some upward modifications in style and price.

... services he desires from the available alternatives. In medical care, however, the patient does not usually make his choice directly. . . . He selects a physician who then makes . . . choices for him.

As mentioned earlier, there does exist some variation in this pattern. For one thing, the degree of activity or control the patient is allowed to assume is related to whether he is consulting a medical practitioner with a "client-dependent" or a "colleague-dependent" practice. In the former instance, the success of the physician (usually a general practitioner, pediatrician, or internist) may depend on the kind of relationship he develops with his patients. As he continues to see and know a patient over a period of time, he may be more inclined to share information with him, give him more control over his treatment sometimes, to the point of yielding to patient demands for medications, hospitalization, and the like.

These client-dependent physicians participate in the professional referral system. The cases they cannot handle are funneled deeper into the medical care system to the specialists — surgeons, neurologists, urologists, radiologists, and the like — whose practices are colleague-dependent. These practitioners, who have no continuing relationship with the patient and see him only on referral, are generally guided almost completely by their medical expertise and not by the patient's demands. This is considered quite desirable by the profession.

The patient, however, usually loses whatever degree of control he may have enjoyed with his primary care practitioner. He is usually sicker, more frightened and overwhelmed, and thus more dependent. The specialist, by virtue of the system, offers the patient very little independence and, generally speaking, interaction is decreased and less open.

The decline in client-dependent practices has resulted in an overall decrease in the input patients have in decisions about their health care. And, even in such practices, the aesculapian concept does not dispose toward sharing information about diagnostic studies, treatment approaches, prognoses, and other data with the patient. His questions go unanswered or are evaded. Obviously, without the necessary data, decision-making and controlling behavior on the part of the patient are ruled out. If he doesn't know that there are other ways in which his problem might be treated, he cannot ask for a different approach, even when the one currently being used turns out to be unsuccessful.

Joint Participation Model

Moving toward the opposite end of the continuum, a model for joint participation emerges. Here, the interaction between physician and patient comes much closer to being one of equals, and decisions are arrived at through a mutual process involving considerable two-way communication.

The influence of the physician will depend not on his power and authority but rather on his persuasive and instructional capacities — on his expertise rather than his authority.

Under these circumstances the patient retains a high degree of control over events that will affect him. Where a surgical procedure seems indicated, for example, the physician makes his informed decision after weighing the feasible alternatives and the risks versus the benefits. Then he provides the patient with the right to undertake a secondary estimation and, in order to help him with this decision, he provides the needed data on other treatment approaches and the likelihood of success.

To arrive at his own decision, the patient must know the physician's preferences, as well as details on how he selects data from his universe of experience. The physician, having made his own decision, attempts to persuade and instruct the patient; but he does not flatly disagree with him, mislead him, bully him, or reject him for a questioning attitude or a final decision that differs from his own. To do so would destroy the collaborative status inherent in the joint participation model.

In situations where the best mode of management is not readily apparent or known by the physician, then patient and physician jointly decide what is best for the patient. An example would be a newly diagnosed diabetic, whose life style, eating patterns, occupation, and other variables should all be considered as the decisions for treatment are made. The search for the answers is part of the therapeutic process.

Pros and Cons

Proponents of the concept of aesculapian authority vehemently argue that this power is quite essential because without it most patients would not undergo the treatment they need. They would be too afraid. Unlike the storekeeper whose success comes from giving his customers what they *want*, physicians must give their clients what they really *need*, which sometimes means giving them what they don't want at all! To accomplish this, the argument goes, control and manipulation of the patient are mandated. Furthermore, supporters of aesculapian authority see the successful wielding of this power as an achievement whereby the patient's normal decision-making abilities are momentarily suspended, much to his own advantage.[6],[7]

Another rationale for the use of aesculapian authority is that the body of medical knowledge is so esoteric and complex that the layman would find it difficult to grasp, much less evaluate, the meaning of his diagnosis and treatment. Because of this presumed ignorance, it is argued, the patient could harm himself if allowed to share in the medical decisions.

Although many patients have undoubtedly been pressured by this awesome authority into accepting the orders of their physicians, the exercise of this aesculapian power has also led to noncompliance. While physicians have been found to underestimate the extent of noncompliance among their patients, studies reveal a rate of 33 to 50 percent.[2] Davis, who

carried out a thorough ___ ___ ,uay .
patient interaction on compliance,   that no)
to attempts by the physician to conti᠊

Other situations found to foster nonco᠊᠊   ᠊᠊᠊ ᠊᠊ occasions when
the physician expresses outright disagreemen᠋ ᠋ .n the patient, when he is
formal and rejecting, and when he fails to provide feedback after extracting
information. It appears, then, that when patients are involved in the
decision-making process, they are most likely to accept the responsibilites
imposed by their condition and go along with the necessary treatment.

How Much Participation?

The question, then, is the relative degree of control to be assumed by both
partners in the transaction. Some physicians involve their clients to the
fullest extent possible in the decision-making process, but others find it
difficult to relinquish control even when it is warranted. Some patients, too,
prefer the passive or "sick" role, finding dependency more acceptable than
the need to make decisions.

Each patient's capabilities and emotional responses will influence the
degree of participation that is appropriate for him. The complexity of the
interaction necessitated by joint participation, for example, would make this
model quite inappropriate for those of low intelligence levels or emotionally
incapable of using their thinking capacities. If the problem has been so
disturbing to the patient that he cannot be rational about it, he is not in a
position to choose what should be done for himself. Similarly, life-
threatening events must be handled with very little or no patient
involvement. On the other hand, if the physician and patient have similiar
educational, intellectual, and experiential backgrounds, and the patient is
psychologically able to deal with the situation at hand he should be allowed
to participate to a much greater extent than is usually the case.

The patient's ability to participate responsibly in the evaluation of the
treatment modes which the physician offers is often underestimated. After
all, the public's knowledge of medicine has grown considerably in the last
fifty years, as has the level of formal education of the populace. Popularized,
self-help medical literature — books, newspaper and magazine articles —
are read avidly these days ("I read about it in the *Reader's Digest*," the patient
tells his physician), and television documentaries and medically-oriented
soap operas all tend to alert the layman to issues of medical care. Therefore,
even when a patient seems to accept the passive, unquestioning role, he may
be harboring serious doubts and misconceptions about the way his
condition is being managed. He hesitates to say so, however.

Beyond this consideration is the detrimental effect that the authoritarian
stance has on the patient's self-concept; it takes away his usual status as a
self-determining adult with reasoning capacity and, above all, human
dignity. The sacrifice of an individual's dignity seems to be an unnecessarily
high price to pay for medical treatment.

It might be said that the patient should be able to resist the authority of a physician if he were motivated to do so, but a number of factors work against the client's developing such an assertive posture. First of all, we are just beginning to learn about human response to authority in general, and some of the recent findings have been both shocking and disillusioning.

In Milgram's landmark studies on man's obedience to authority, individuals were commanded by an experimenter to administer electric shocks of increasing severity to protesting, possibly endangered, victims. Most of the subjects obeyed the authority figure in spite of the fact that the direct action conflicted with their fundamental standards of morality. The author explains, "The key to the behavior of the subject lies not in pent-up anger or aggression but in the nature of their relationship to authority. They have given themselves to authority."[11]

In short, few people were found to have the resources needed to resist authority. Then, when we remember the potency of physician authority, we can readily see the difficulty a patient would have in resisting such power. In addition, the patient has a strong desire to be accepted, liked, and cared for by the physician and a deep fear of being rejected, which stems from his enforced and very real dependency on the physician. He hesitates to disagree, to assert himself.

Patients' Rights

In a free society such as ours there is the philosophical question of individual rights. Basically, I believe that the issue of what is good for the individual is an issue that only he can determine. Immediate threats to life are the obvious exception. Furthermore, the fact that a client has made a choice of professional services does not mean that he has forever relinquished his right to participate in the decision-making process and to be informed of significant alternatives in diagnosis and treatment. He also retains the right to withdraw from the service if he so desires.

The whole concept of patients' rights is fairly new. Yet, gradually, there has been a rise in client demands, evidenced primarily in the escalation of lawsuits against physicians, nurses, and health care agencies. "Informed consent" for procedures has become a legal issue of growing magnitude. Prior to the early 1960s the decision to perform a medical procedure belonged to the physician alone. Since that time a number of court decisions have clearly and firmly established the patient's right of "self-determination." In a recent article in the *Journal of the American Medical Association* on this subject, Don H. Mills remarks:

He (the patient) cannot, of course, decide whether the procedure is adequately indicated, for that requires more medical expertise than he possesses. But once he is told that the procedure is recommended, he then must have enough information to decide whether the hoped-for benefits are, in his eyes, sufficient to risk the possible hazards.[12]

Mills goes on to explore just how far the physician must go in listing hazards. He suggests a middle-of-the-road approach that would be "both consistent with good medical care and that affords reasonable legal safety."

He never explains why full information disclosed to the patient would be antithetic to "good medical care," but this surely stems from the belief that the patient would be too afraid to undergo the procedure if he were acquainted with the potential dangers.

But, counterbalancing the presumed fear, what degree of rage may result when a patient does suffer a complication and has had no forewarning of the possibility and no part in the decision to take that risk? Consider, for example, the physician who recommends a simple mastectomy to a woman with breast cancer but fails to tell her that a modified radical or a radical mastectomy is another approach. I believe he has done his patient a great disservice. She has the right to decide whether the increased hazards or the degree of bodily disfigurement are worth even a small hope of greater success. Moreover, according to a study by Hershey and Bushkoff, disclosures to the patient did *not* cause clients to withhold their consent for procedures.[13]

A Personal Experience

It was when my own need for medical care arose that I learned so much about the character and effects of physician-patient relationships. My physician first interacted with me in a highly authoritarian way but, fortunately, our relationship soon developed into one that was highly facilitative and essentially based on joint participation. The difference that the two approaches made in my feelings of self-esteem and control, and thus my ability to cope with the crisis at hand, was marked.

As my illness and hospitalization began, I followed along in the usual way with what my physician ordered. I had no reason not be be compliant. Relief from pain was my foremost need. It was after the x-rays and other diagnostic tests were completed and the physician recommended surgery that I began to resist his controlling behavior. Over the telephone our conversation went as follows:

DOCTOR: Your gall bladder didn't visualize again today.

PATIENT: I know!

DOCTOR: You do? I think we should take you to surgery tomorrow *(warmly)*.

PATIENT: I'm not ready for *that.*

DOCTOR: Well, we work for you! *(assertively)*

PATIENT: But I haven't had any symptoms before *(voice shrinking)*.

DOCTOR: You can have a perforated ulcer without any symptoms, too!

PATIENT: *(sighing heavily)* Does it have to be done now? This is not a good time for me.

DOCTOR: If you come back to me in two weeks, I would tell you the same thing. You're sitting on a loaded pistol! *(aggressively)*

This interchange continued for a while longer, with him dictating to me from his position of authority. He was the parent and I the dependent, deferent, acquiescing child.

This physician obviously uses authoritarianism with considerable success, and his actions undoubtedly stem from a well-intentioned belief that his patients' welfares are at stake. Surgeons may rely more heavily on this interaction model than other medical practitioners, because surgery tends to create more stress and anxiety in the patient than other methods of treatment. For me, though, the approach was devastating because I felt as if my usual identity as a self-determining adult was being replaced with that of a dependent, passive, and helpless non-being. This altered self-image was quite unacceptable; the result was feelings of anxiety, frustration, and anger.

The physician expected a child-like, unquestioning faith and trust, and I found myself unable to meet his expectations. True, I respected his abilities as a highly competent clinician and surgeon and felt physically safe in his care; this made it all the more difficult to resist his authority. But that wasn't enough. I wanted full access to the data and reasoning upon which he made his decision. Furthermore, I believed that I was in the best position to decide whether or not to undergo surgery at that time. I needed his help to make that decision, however. And I also needed to know that he saw me as an individual rather than just "another cholecystectomy."

While I was able to put up some passive resistance to his demands, it surprises me that I was not more openly aggressive in my interaction with him. In fact, as he became more dominant, I became less assertive and more passive. In normal situations, my response is just the opposite. My reaction was certainly not due to the fact that he was a physician *per se*, because over the year I had established too many professional co-equal relationships with physicians to be impressed by that fact. Instead, I attribute my response to the awesome power physicians exercise over their patients: I was no exception.

Two or three hours after our telephone conversation, the physician appeared in person. He had made the trip to help me with my decision, and his approach was entirely different this time. He provided me with much of the basis for his decision and when I decided against surgery for the time being, he said, "All right, that's fine," obviously genuine in his acceptance of me.

I remember being quite surprised and puzzled by the decided contrast in his behavior. In the next few days our relationship continued to develop according to the latter interaction pattern, and my confidence in him grew immeasurably. Eventually I decided to have surgery. Although I was moved to this decision both by the continuation of pain and by the passage of enough time to work through the shock and denial phases of my illness, I am absolutely certain that I would have continued to reject surgery if I had not had the benefit of the ensuing therapeutic relationship with my physician.

Before I felt safe enough to relinquish all control of myself and my destiny to the physician, I had to believe that he cared what happened to me and valued my existence as an individual. The extensive help he provided me in making the decision for surgery went a long way toward convincing me that he did, indeed, value me as an individual. In addition, his interaction with me immediately before the surgery, even when I was already in the operating room, was extremely reassuring — more so than I would have predicted. His evident concern apparently represented the much needed validation that I was still a person (even in that setting) and not just a "gall bladder."

Implications For the Nurse

This discussion has centered on the dynamics of the patient-physician relationship and has explored a phenomenon, labeled aesculapian authority, that usually goes unnoticed, but nonetheless plays a highly significant role in the health care delivery system. An understanding of the phenomenon should help the nurse to improve both the system and her nursing care.

First of all, the nurse is in a key position to help both the patient and his family deal effectively with problems they may be experiencing, either in their relationship with the physician or with the advice he has given them. As with other problems, the patient needs the benefits of facilitative communication. Yet many nurses become extremely anxious when a patient alludes in any way to negative feelings about a physician — or another nurse, for that matter. Many times the nurse rushes to protect the physician: "You have an excellent doctor." This effectively blocks further communications on the subject and makes it even more difficult for the patient to exercise his decision-making powers.

The hospitalized patient is literally an inmate of a total institution, wholly dependent on the nurses for care and cut off from the usual sources of information and social support needed to assume an active role in making decisions. It is not uncommon for the staff to intimidate the patient in subtle ways or to exercise covert threats of rejection to get him to go along with what the physician and nurse dictate. The nurse's actions sometime stem from her feelings of subordination to the physician. She may actually fear rejection by him or retributive measures. Instead of seeing herself as a patient advocate, she sees herself as a physician helper. It is more rewarding or less threatening for her to please the physician than it is to meet the needs of the patient.

This does not imply in any way that the nurse should feel that she must protect the patient *from* the physician. I say this because I have known a number of nurses who have adopted this stance as a defensive response to physician dominance. Even though the patient may have difficulty confronting or communicating with the physician, he usually doesn't need or want protection from him. What he does need is the opportunity to talk about his concerns with a genuine, warm, and empathic helper who will help him to work out his own solutions.

It should be pointed out that the patient is not too likely to think of the nurse in this way. He probably feels that his physician is the only person that he can count on to take care of him on a continuing basis and be concerned with his needs over time. With the prevailing nursing care system, the patient receives care from innumerable nurses during hospitalization, and rarely do opportunities exist for in-depth, continuing relationships. Primary nursing is an exciting departure from the traditional system and promises to go a long way toward improving this situation.[14]

Offering advice and opinions is not appropriate, as is true in all instances of therapeutic communication. Moreover, the nurse is obviously not in a position to advise about medical decisions. It is the physician's responsibility to present the patient with his medical opinion and the data he bases it on, although the nurse should assume responsibility for clarifying any misconceptions on the patient's part of a physician's explanations. Primarily, however, she helps the patient to work through his feelings by means of a helping relationship based on a high level of empathy. Knowledge of the phenomenon described here should offer valuble data for this empathic interaction.[15]

As a patient, I was fortunate to have this kind of help. On only one occasion did a nurse argue with a decision I had made. Several nurses, however, erred in the other direction, for it is equally unwise to agree, unreservedly on all occasions, with a patient's point of view. As Rogers explains:

> In almost every phase of our lives . . . we find ourselves under the rewards and punishments of external judgments . . . But in my experience they do not make for personal growth, and hence I do not believe that they are a part of a helping relationship. Curiously enough, a positive evaluation is as threatening in the long run as a negative one, since to inform someone that he is good implies that you also have the right to tell him he is bad. So I have come to feel that the more I can keep a relationship free of judgment and evaluation, the more this will permit the other person to reach the point where he recognizes that the locus of evaluation, the center of responsibility, lies within himself. The meaning and value of his experience is in the last analysis something which is up to him, and no amount of external judgment can alter this.[16]

Decisions, then, to be good ones for the individual making the choice, should emanate solely from within that person.

As has been pointed out, one of the key ways to keep patients from exercising control is to restrict the information they receive. Throughout my years of practice, I have made it a habit to do just the opposite; while this generally goes against established policies, I believe that is quite essential for the nurse to break down the barriers. As a patient, I wanted to know my vital signs, the drugs I was being given, the results of diagnostic tests, and all other data on my "case." To get this information, I usually had to ask for it, sometime with quite a bit of determination and forcefulness in my voice.

In other words, nurses and other health team members weren't in the habit of volunteering this information and sometimes felt quite uncomfortable in doing so. I got my share of stylized responses such as "Your temperature is fine." I didn't want reassurance; I wanted exact information. In one instance, a staff nurse brought in a new medication and when I asked what it was, she responded, "I can't tell you! You of all people should know that!" That made me angry, even though I knew I could ask another nurse who would tell me. It seemed illogical, indeed, that this nurse had the right to know more about my treatment than I did myself.

After surgery a nurse colleague who was taking care of me let me look at the pathology report. This was very reassuring, not because I would have doubted her truthfulness if she had told me the results, but because she was allowing me to exercise my usual way of assessing a patient — this time, myself. All the concrete knowledge I had about myself increased my feelings of power and control as well as my self-esteem.

There are a few patients who definitely do not want this kind of information; they are less anxious if they assume a position of blind dependence. Then, again, many people may not *seem* to want to know; when questioned, however, they express a deep-felt desire to be informed, but say they "didn't feel" that it was their right. Therefore, it is absolutely essential for the nurse to make keen assessments as to each patient's needs and capabilities.

More Than One Villain

Physicians are not the only ones to exercise acsculapian authority. Nurses are often authoritarian, too, so, while medicine has been singled out here, it is little more of a villain than nursing. The pervasiveness of the medical model accounts for some of this behavior; however, it seems to me that the nurse sometimes uses her authority to build up her professional status as well. How often, for instance, is the patient allowed to participate in decisions about his nursing care? Here is where the nurse can considerably enhance the patient's sense of control, by encouraging him to participate in innumerable decisions, ranging from whether or not he will have a public health nurse referral to the determination of the time of his treatments and medications.

As is true in medical management, the nurse who allows the patient to participate in these decisions runs the risk that he will choose an alternative that she does not believe to be in his best interest. If attempts to instruct and persuade the patient fail, then the nurse must have enough humility to allow him the greater value of the dignity of his own choice. If she imposes her own notion of what is good onto the patient, she will at the same time reduce his dignity.

In Retrospect

An unexpected encounter with hospitalization and surgery has prompted this attempt to provide some insight into the almost mystical relationship between physicians and patients. Half-gods, physicians resemble. Yet for patients to acquiesce completely with this concept, without demanding some reasonable degree of participation in the decision-making, seems unreasonable. Certainly this whole process, especially as it relates to the third party in the person of the nurse, deserves much more attention than it has received.

In the same play from which I quoted at the beginning of this article is the following exchange:

DOCTOR. Take again your bed, sir;
Sleep is a sovereign physic.
ANTONINUS. Take an ass's head, sir:
Confusion on your fooleries, your charms!
Thy pills and base apothecary drugs
Threaten'd to bring unto me? Out, you imposter!
Quacksalving, cheating mountebank! Your skill
Is to make sound men sick, and sick men kill.[17]

Strong language, perhaps, and medicine has come a long way in the over
350 years that have passed since those words were spoken. Nevertheless,
today's society is more and more an outspoken and critical one — one that
demands to *know*, rather than just be *told*. An unresponsive, dictatorial
attitude on the part of either physician or nurse is increasingly likely
to evoke a reaction that could strongly resemble that of Antoninus — three
centuries later.

FOOTNOTES

1. Gifford, W., ed. W. Bulmer and Co., 1813, p. 76.
2. Duff, R. S. and Hollingshead, A. B. *Sickness and Society*, New York,
   Harper & Row, 1968, p. 382.
3. Paterson, T. T. *Management Theory*. London, Business Publications,
   1966.
4. Siegler, Miriam, and Osmond, Humphrey. Aesculapian authority.
   Hastings Center Studies 1(2):41-52, 1973.
5. Feldstein, P. J. Research on the demand for health services.
   Milbank Mem.Fund Q. 44(Suppl): 138, July 1966.
6. Paterson, *op.cit.*
7. Siegler and Osmond, *op.cit.*
8. Davis, M. S. Variations in patients' compliance with doctors'
   advice. *Am. J. Public Health* 58:274-288,Feb. 1968.
9. *Ibid.*
10. Davis, M. S., and von der Lippe, R. P. Discharge from hospital
    against medical advice: a study of reciprocity in the doctor-patient
    relationship. *Soc.Sci.Med.* 1:336-342, 1968.
11. Milgram, Stanley. *Obedience to Authority: An Experimental View*. New
    York, Harper & Row, 1973, p. 168.
12. Mills, D. H. Whither informed consent? *JAMA* 229:307, July
    15, 1974.
13. Hershey, Nathan, and Bushkoff, S. H. *Informed Consent
    Study*. Pittsburgh, Aspen Systems Corp., 1969.
14. Marram, G. D., and others. *Primary Nursing: A Model for Individualized
    Care*. St. Louis, C. V. Mosby Co., 1974.
15. Kalisch, B. J. What is empathy? *Am.J.Nurs.* 73:1548-1552,
    Sept. 1973.
16. Rogers, C. R. The characteristics of a helping relationship.
    Personnel Guid.J. 27:6-15, Sept. 1958.
17. Gifford, *op.cit.*, p. 78.

The Erosion of Professional Authority: A Cross-Cultural Inquiry in the Case of the Physician

Marie R. Haug

Theoretical Issues

One of the phenomena which seems increasingly to characterize relationships between professionals and their clients in the United States is an unwillingness on the part of the client to accept without question the authority of the professional. The "revolt of the client" (Haug and Sussman, 1969), and the demand for accountability (Reiff, 1971) signify a growing public suspicion that neither the expertise nor the good will of the professional are to be taken on trust, at face value. While this trend can be observed in the United States, having been noted by writers with respect to medicine as well as other professional fields (Reeder, 1972; Eulau, 1973; Haug, 1975), its occurrence in other parts of the world with differing social, cultural and economic structures and various divisions of labor in the human services, has not yet been systematically studied. The research outlined in these pages represents a preliminary attempt to determine the nature and extent of this phenomenon in the case of the physician, in two different societies, the United Kingdom and the U.S.S.R. Utilizing a sociological perspective, the study explores the basis of primary care physician authority in the context of two types of socialized delivery system of medical care. The aim is to identify those societal characteristics as well as those individual characteristics of patients and physicians which affect the authority relationship in these diverse national contexts.

Most sociologists in the United States have modeled their definitions of profession on the historic trio of medicine, law, and the clergy, focusing on the command of an esoteric body of knowledge acquired through academic training, and a service orientation, which account both for professional freedom from lay control, i.e., autonomy in work performance, and socially sanctioned power over clients, i.e., authority in the practitioner-client relationship. According to this view, it is the professions' monopoly over knowledge not easily accessible to the public, coupled with a claim to a public service outlook, which legitimates the professional's authority in dealing with clients, and institutionalizes client obligations to trust the professional and comply with his prescriptions (Moore, 1970). Even those who have argued that profession is essentially a folk concept (Becker,

From *The Milbank Memorial Fund Quarterly/Health and Society,* Vol. 54, No. 1, Winter 1976. By permission of the author and publisher.

1962) concede that knowledge claims undergird professionals' work autonomy and client acceptance of their authority. In fact it has been suggested that the presence or absence of this power position is what distinguishes professions from non-professions (Freidson, 1970). The sick-role concept (Parsons, 1951), the most widely used sociological interpretation of the doctor-patient relationship, is a derivative of the theory of professions: it is the obligation of the sick to seek expert help in order to get well, and thus to defer to the physician's professional authority. The "competence" gap between doctor and patient justifies the asymmetrical power relationship and the patient's trust, confidence, and norm of obedience.

Implicit in the focus on professional autonomy is the likelihood of conflict with the authority structure of bureaucratic organizations, in which professional work is increasingly located. Indeed, the literature on this topic has been voluminous in recent years (Perrow, 1972), However, the strain between the two power bases may currently be more imagined than actual. In fact, professions often in practice forge a partnership with bureaucracy in organizational work settings, in order to buttress their relations with clients (Freidson, 1970). In this case, the bureaucratic rules and regulations are used to enforce professional decisions with respect to client actions, whether or not the client has accepted the value stricture that it is in his best interests to comply.

Given these multiple pressures on the client to conform, how does it happen that both the autonomy and authority of the professional are nevertheless being challenged, at least in this country? Explanations for the American phenomenon have been sought in the erosion of the professional's monopoly over knowledge, the sophistication attending rising educational levels of the general public, and new divisions of labor which redistribute expertise in the human service field. Changes in control over esoteric knowledge, as its storage and retrieval are computerized, present a potential threat to the eroding monopoly. Furthermore, aggregation of clients in bureaucratic settings may have the unanticipated consequence of stimulating a form of "client consciousness" of their common fate, leading to social movements which challenge professional power and demand accountability for practitioners' actions (Haug, 1973; 1974).

It is apparent that these developments apply to the physician in the United States. Popular knowledge of health issues is disseminated by the media; health organizations urge people to watch for signs of cancer or heart disease; Dr. Spock is only one of a range of do-it-yourself medical guides, of which a more recent example is *Our Bodies Our Selves* (Boston Women's Health Book Collective, 1973); patients with chronic conditions are trained for self-care; and the fact that the majority of the adult American public has completed more than 12 years of schooling (U.S. Bureau of the Census, 1972: 111) implies not only some basic education in nutrition and hygiene but also potential for skepticism about others' knowledge claims (Wilensky, 1964). The computerization of many aspects of medical services is already an established fact (Schwartz, 1970).

As for changes in the division of labor, these also are characteristic of the medical profession. The extent to which tasks of the physician are gradually being given to paraprofessionals or to those now claiming to be professionals in their own right is well documented (Lefkowitz and Ausmus, 1970). Babies are delivered by a midwife with specialized training, and the nurse-clinician handles many aspects of infant and child care; the intensive-care-unit nurse deals with postoperative crises, and the physician's assistant takes over tasks previously performed by a doctor. One prominent physician educator has suggested that by 1980 physician's assistants or technicians will be setting simple fractures and taking out appendixes (Geiger, 1972: 109).

A complexity which is most marked in medicine is the sexual division of labor. In the United States, the most powerful role, that of the physician, is largely in male hands, while most persons to whom former physician tasks have devolved, as a result of the change in the division of labor, are female. To the extent that societal values produce differences in acceptance of autonomy and authority on the basis of the sex of the authority figure, this confounds an estimate of the effect of the new occupational mix on patient responses to the claims of expertise.

Moreover, physicians are not immune to the loss of autonomy inherent in demands for accountability, and public rather than peer evaluation. The evidence for this development is more tenuous, and it may be related to factors in addition to schooling increments and the changing labor mix. Thus the well-documented increases in malpractice suits may spring at least in part from a general consumerism ideology. On the other hand, proposed legislation to monitor physician use of human subjects in medical research has political overtones. Organized patient movements for improvements in hospital ambulatory clinic care challenge physician control of service delivery at the institutional level, and offer a portent of future developments when patient care is dispensed in a bureaucratized setting. Each of these is in its own way a sign that the doctor's dictum is not necessarily taken as the last word.[1]

In sum, it is suggested here that profound change in authority relations is occurring in which knowledge is losing its role as a power base as it becomes demonopolized, and that the medical profession may be viewed as a prototype of this trend.

Research Question and Method of Data Collection

But is this an emergent phenomenon peculiar to the United States? Is the professional authority model applicable cross-culturally? Specifically, is physician medical knowledge the explanation for this occupation's legitimated power over patients under varying societal conditions, or are there other factors which structure the doctor-patient relationship? Derivative questions address whether variations in patient acceptance of medical-practitioner authority occur by (a) various *individual* characteristics, for example, level of patient education; and (b) various *societal* characteristics, for example, bureaucratic structure.

Data relevant to these research questions have been collected through informal interviews conducted by the author with medical practitioners and knowledgeable informants in Great Britain and the U.S.S.R. during the winter and spring of 1974. The focus was on general practice, as offering the widest range of physician-public interactions. Great Britain and the U.S.S.R. were selected for study because they varied from each other and from the United States on a number of major parameters.

Although both offer a form of socialized medicine, in Great Britain primary care is still dispensed largely by solo practitioners or small group practices, while the Soviet system provides care in large centers or polyclinics. Educational levels and the sexual division of medical labor in Great Britain are more similar to the situation in the United States, while fewer average years of schooling and a predominantly female medical profession characterize the U.S.S.R. Finally, the British and American concepts of profession are virtually identical, whereas the Soviets have no comparable definition; in fact the Russian language does not even have a word for profession in our sense, using the term "intelligentsia" for a more general category.

There was no attempt at random sampling of interviewees. Instead a *purposive* sample was selected, taking into account geographic location and position in the health delivery system. In Britain key respondents were chosen on the advice of British social scientists knowledgeable about their country's health system, and practitioners of varying ideological stance. From this beginning a "snowballing" technique was used, in which respondents were selected from persons recommended by those already interviewed as having information germane to the study, including those with different perspectives. In all, 47 persons, including 15 physicians in general practice, were formally interviewed.

In the U.S.S.R., heads of medical facilities were selected on the basis of their availability for interview as determined by Intourist, the official tourist agency. Eleven physicians, in seven polyclinics from Leningrad to Tblisi, were among the 22 interviewed. In both Britain and the Soviet Union, respondents were secured from several geographic areas, and from academic medical figures as well as from active practitioners.

All interviews were reconstructed on tape immediately after the interview, using field notes and recollections. Although the interviews were informal and unstructured, they followed a general format which began with a question about the current characteristics of doctor-patient relationsips from the interviewee's perspective, followed by inquiries about recent changes, if any, in the nature of that interaction. Questions about the effect of age, education, and occupation of the patients on the relationship were included, as well as probes about those persons considered easiest and most difficult to treat, and why.

In both the U.S.S.R. and Great Britain the data are chiefly from a medical practitioner's perspective, since no patients' organizations as such were found in the U.S.S.R., and only limited contact was possible in Great Britain with two existing groups, themselves circumscribed in scope. Despite this shortcoming, it was possible to gather indications of developments relevant to the research questions posed and thus with impact on theories of professions, and derivatively on doctor-patient relationships in the sick role.

Research Findings

Several themes emerged from these experiences. First, on a general level, physician authority is currently being challenged, and this phenomenon is by no means idiosyncratic to the United States. Moreover, from the physician's perspective, in both Great Britain and the U.S.S.R., professional authority in the physician-patient relationship varies with patient education, but patient age also is an important variable. In both countries, despite the differences in the bureaucratization of the medical care delivery systems, health practitioners have similar gatekeeper roles from which they derive power over patients not directly related to their medical expertise, since physicians control access to many non-medical benefits valued by the public. An unexpected finding is the overriding importance of historical developments, cultural traditions, and ideology in explaining the position accorded physicians in the division of labor and public acceptance of their authority. The specific impact of the discovery and the development of technological aids of various kinds is only one of these factors, along with the effects of war, social-class history, and the sex of the practitioner. Each of these themes suggests, from different perspectives, the changing role of knowledge monopoly, and the extent to which factors other than knowledge undergird professional power in general and physician authority in particular.

INDIVIDUAL CHARACTERISTICS: THE AGE VARIABLE

In Great Britain, several informants suggested that older patients are more willing to accept the physician's authority because they are grateful for the "free" medical care, remembering the period before World War II when the fee-for-service system existed and care was beyond the reach of many. As one Welsh physician commented, some of the elderly are very respectful and deferential, "excusing themselves for bothering the doctor, bringing gifts of boxes of chocolates at Christmas, or half a dozen eggs during the year."[2] On the other hand, another general practitioner, in a Midlands health center, had noted the disaffection of some older patients who "expected the doctor to drop in and have a cup of tea and a chat," as in an earlier, more leisurely time, and were upset when this did not occur. In general, however, British health workers considered the older patients more accepting of the physician's authority than the younger, who, many felt, tend to argue, question, and reject authority. The explanation offered, it should be noted, was not only a habit of deference among the elderly, but the experiences of this age cohort from a period prior to the establishment of the National Health Service.

In the U.S.S.R. age was also viewed as a meaningful variable, but with a somewhat different focus. Some physicians felt, in the words of one informant, that "the aged, when they are ill, are eager to be cured and so carry out all instructions as carefully as possible, while with the young people it is just the opposite — they refuse to obey." Another theme was more dominant — that the elderly are more demanding, questioning, and unwilling to bow to the doctor's orders. Since they are not working, not busy, they come in more often for small matters, although usually all they need is reassurance. As one woman general practitioner put it, "The retired who have grandchildren to care for do not come as frequently, but if they are not working and have nothing to do, they read *Health,* a popular magazine, or medical columns in the paper, or listen to radio and TV, and come in asking for one pill or another, or insist that they have symptoms requiring medication, or just because they want a social visit with the doctor." Since the primary health care system in the U.S.S.R. is based on a network of regional or neighborhood "polyclinics," easily accessible, at least in the city, to would-be patients without charge, the structural arrangements facilitate "over-utilization" coupled with challenges of the physician's advice.

Variation in acceptance of professional authority by client age cohort is congruent with a model of profession based on the occupational characteristic of knowledge monopoly to the extent that the age variable is related to educational level and thus to differential breakdown of that monopoly. Indeed, in the U.S.S.R. this relationship is made explicit. It is because the old have time and inclination to read and listen to health education materials that they develop knowledge claims of their own and challenge the word of the doctor.

INDIVIDUAL CHARACTERISTICS: THE EDUCATION VARIABLE

Education of the client as a critical factor in eroding professional authority emerged clearly in both countries studied, although in Britain it was often expressed in social-class terms, whereas in the U.S.S.R. the differences were formulated in terms of schooling and health education, as well as non-manual versus manual categories. One eminent general practitioner in London pointed out that middle- and upper-class patients are more critical than working-class patients. For them, he commented "the knowledge and skill of the general practitioner in terms of his present training is not too much unlike their own sophistication because they also have university degrees." A Midlands physician said he preferred local poor people, because they are "grateful for any help; but couldn't stand Londoners and middle-class types," who were full of questions and arguments. Indeed a thread ran through many of the British interviews, that patients were growing more knowledgeable, demanding more explanations, and in this sense, for some doctors, becoming more difficult, i.e., less willing to accept authority, a finding congruent with data reported by Mechanic (1970) from an earlier study of a larger sample.

In the Soviet Union, a similar theme was expressed by several polyclinic physicians. As one remarked, "it is much easier to treat manual workers as patients. The intelligentsia and the non-manual workers are educated. They read books, literature, listen to radio, watch TV; when they speak of an illness they give not only the symptoms but also the diagnosis. It is easier for the doctor if the patient does not try to tell the doctor what to do." On another occasion, during a group interview, a male doctor had said that it was necessary to explain everything to neurotic patients because they want to know everything. The researcher then probed about the effect of education and asked, apropos of the fact that the Soviet state had recently set compulsory education at 10 years, what would happen when all Soviet citizens had a university education. The head of the clinic, a woman physician, laughed, and said that "then all patients will be neurotic, there will be much work for the doctor, lots of arguments and different kinds of diseases to deal with."

There was, however, a striking difference between the U.S.S.R. and Great Britain on the education variable. In the U.S.S.R. there was heavy constant emphasis on teaching patients about health matters. Every polyclinic had posters and displays in hallways and waiting rooms about nutrition, hygiene, exercise, care of chronic conditions, infant development, and the like. Available in waiting rooms were varicolored illustrated folders on specific diseases and treatment, some with diagrams of various organs to explain the purposes of medical procedures. In several polyclinics the researcher noticed that physical therapy rooms had large wall displays with photographs of each piece of equipment along with statements of their purpose and benefits. In each facility visited there was an office responsible for fostering patient education, although much of the material was obviously centrally prepared. The mecical staff was well aware of the dilemma involved in educating patients while at the same time preferring them to accept the physician's advice without question. Several explained that the education material focused on treatment, rather than symptoms, because if there was too much information about symptoms, the polyclinic might have an excess of patients with imaginary ailments. On the other hand, some others suggested that a few early symptoms were specified, and not too much about treatment, to encourage consultation with a physician.

There was one point on which doctors in both countries firmly agreed, and that was that patients should *not* have access to their own medical records. As one doctor in the U.S.S.R. put it, "patients should *not*, of course, know everything," echoing a general practitioner in Great Britain who responded emphatically in response to an inquiry about patients' seeing their files, "That's stupid . . . ignorance is bliss for most." The implication was clear that knowledge should not extend to the point where it would be painful to a person. For the patient's own protection, the doctors agreed, there were some things that only they should know. The paradox in this view was understood by a Soviet cancer specialist, who wondered how patients could be persuaded to trust their doctors, and believe what they were told, when at the same time it is common knowledge that doctors may fail to tell cancer victims what their diagnosis is, or even lie about it.

SOCIETAL CHARACTERISTICS: DOCTORS AS BUREAUCRATIC GATEKEEPERS

The gatekeeper role of the physician emerged as a reinforcement of medical power under the British National Health Service as well as the Soviet medical system. In Britain, general practitioners must sign "certificates" which validate illness claims and thus a person's right to paid sick leave if he is off work for more than three days. One informant noted that just before the 1974 miners' strike, surgeries and hospital casualty departments in Wales were flooded with patients — miners claiming they were sick in order to get social security payments during the strike. Many physicians are annoyed by certification duties because they view this as essentially nonmedical dirty work, in which the task involves striking a bargain with the worker as to how much of the desired time off is reasonably justified. In some cases this bargaining job has been sloughed off on nurse or receptionist, but the doctor's signature is still needed on the form. The physician's work is also critical in getting in a priority for an elderly patient in "council housing," the publicly supported dwellings for the aged and needy, or a telephone installed for an old or sick person living alone. In rural areas or smaller communities the doctor is still presumed to know people on his patient roster well enough to sign gun-license applications or provide character references for young job hunters.

The British general practitioner's control over access to values in the medical arena is also a buttress to his authority, and indeed one protection against encroachments from paraprofessionals. He provides the only entry through the public system to hospitals, and the consultants, or specialists, located there. He is the only channel to medications on prescription - only lists, such as the barbiturates and tranquilizers. Some practitioners indicated that a large part of their practice consisted of prescribing these drugs to individuals with personal and emotional problems. One unpublished study shows that more than half the British practitioners surveyed believe from one third to two thirds of their consultations have a psychogenic component, and four out of five estimate that 80 percent or more of their patients arrive at the surgery expecting a prescription.[3] One physician interviewed estimated that nearly half of his consultations involved psychosocial problems, anxiety, and depression, often of women patients, both young and middle aged, who would come in for tranquilizers.

If the doctor tries to deny the prescription the patient will say, "I've got to have them. I can't cope. The children are getting on my nerves," and feeling the patient is in a state, the doctor gives the prescription.

In the U.S.S.R., the medical system is the gatekeeper not only for paid absences from work, but also for continuation on the job, as well as side benefits such as special vacation privileges. The general practitioner in the regional polyclinic certifies workers for sick leave and approves pay for illness. More than this, in order to stay on the job, whether in production industry or in a white-collar enterprise, workers must receive an annual, or in some cases, a semi-annual, medical checkup. They must show their "card" at the enterprise to prove that they have complied with this requirement in order to continue employment. These examinations are often given at the "enterprise polyclinic," an all-purpose primary and chronic care medical center attached to large establishments such as factories, merchandising complexes, or universities. These enterprise polyclinics, as distinct from the regional polyclinics which are based on neighborhood subdivisions, also have the special gatekeeper role of deciding which workers will be able to take advantage of the health resorts, spas, and vacation facilities run by the enterprise union. Since space is limited, and the benefits of cut-rate prices at desirable vacation locations are much sought after, the physician's gatekeeper role and attendant authority is by no means inconsiderable. Notably in the U.S.S.R., as in Great Britain, sick-leave certificates and other similar gatekeeper functions are based on striking a bargain with the applicant, in order to maintain the patient's good will and cooperation for the future, and not solely on medical criteria or professional expertise.

SOCIETAL CHARACTERISTICS: TECHNOLOGY AND AUTHORITY

Still another pervasive theme, but stressed mainly in the British data, is the modified role of the medical professional as a result of historical changes in conceptions of the nature of health and illness, following in part from the discovery of new drugs and therapies and the invention of medical technologies, tests, and diagnostic and treatment devices. As one general practitioner in London put it, "There has been a profound change in the last twenty years . . . The person sees himself as ill at an earlier stage and with fewer symptoms . . . It is an age in which people are not willing to tolerate anxiety or minor symptoms; they want alterations in their experience of life and they turn to the general practitioner," who has been forced to change his attitudes. "His apostolic function has been reduced. No longer can he say, 'I'm the doctor, do as I tell you.' Now there is a transaction, with the outcomes the result of a collusive effort." Another physician, in a Midlands medical center, also remarked that the concept of illness and medicine has changed, but focused on drug discoveries during and after World War II as explanation. Before that, "doctors had only a bedside manner, colored water, and aspirin." Now patients know about the new magic of pills and technical procedures, and demand that these services be made available by the doctor. In fact several informants noted that patient requests to be referred for diagnostic tests, as carried out in hospitals, were a way of rejecting the authority of the physician in favor of the authority of technology. And a nursing officer commented that godlike tests were replacing the godlike physician as a subject for obeisance and belief.

Only passing references to these developments appear in the Soviet data, and when they do, the perspective is different. Instead of tests substituting for the authority of the primary care physician they are viewed as reinforcing it. Several polyclinic chiefs announced with pride that their staff had a perfect record — all diagnoses made by the general practitioners without the benefit of the technical apparatus available in hospitals and specialty clinics, have been validated by the tests of the specialists. One chief pointed out that the way new doctors in the clinic gained authority was by having their diagnoses and treatment plans coincide with the recommendation of the hospital specialists.

Thus while new medicines and technologies were seen by practitioners in both countries as affecting doctor-patient relationships, the direction of the effect vis-à-vis professional authority was conceptualized in different ways. The findings suggest that various aspects of a physician's tasks differentially affect his authority image. Uncertain diagnosis diminishes, whereas verified diagnosis enhances, that image.

SOCIETAL CHARACTERISTICS: HISTORY, CULTURE, AND IDEOLOGY

Medical history is only one among the set of variables found to affect the physician-client relationship; other historical, cultural, and ideological forces also shape, and perhaps even determine, the meaning of the professional category in division of labor in these two countries.

In Great Britain, there were repeated references to these factors as of critical importance, particularly with respect to the general practitioner, whose *need* for clinical knowledge and whose *command* of psychosocial knowledge were both seen as limited. One prominent general practitioner said of his colleagues that perhaps the quip was true: they are overtrained for what they do and undertrained for what they are supposed to do. Their authority, then, comes from sources other than body of knowledge.

The most salient supportive factor is the aristocratic tradition, which still casts its aura over medicine. Despite the absorption of lower-class apothecaries and barbers into the occupation of physician and surgeon, the status of the upper-class incumbents remains dominant. As more than one informant pointed out, until fairly recently, upper-class families expected the oldest son to take over the estate, the second son to enter the clergy, and the third son to become a physician. All went to a university, and this fact, more than the specific skills acquired, distinguished them from the common folk, who in the class system in Britain were expected to respect and defer to their betters. In some back-country sections of Scotland and Wales, patients still stand when they come in to see the doctor, and actually or symbolically "touch their forelocks." The giving of gifts at Christmas is another manifestation of this habit of deference.

Furthermore, part of the aristocratic tradition is the lord's obligation for public service, a carryover of the feudal value system in which the lord was presumed to have the best interests of his poor and ignorant serfs at heart. The claim that medicine has scientifically based curative power is a relatively new basis for physician authority, and is grafted onto the earlier and more internalized public belief that the doctor's social position merits faith and compliance. Thus as one informant declared, "Doctors are living on the trust engendered from the earlier model of the physician." And another noted that the doctor's ability to secure non-medical services, like better housing and a telephone, is a hangover from "the old days when their word counted for a lot because of their upper-class position rather than their medical status."

An interacting trend is the spreading ideology of collectivism and socialism in Britain. This orientation contains the notion of obedience, the value of deferring to the common good, and the belief that authority should flow to the experts who have the common good at heart. A curious anomaly is that this belief structure also puts physicians in the role of public servants, whose training is paid for by the public and whose services are a public right. Thus the general practitioner should always be available, night and day, to anyone who asks for his attention. The outcome of this mix of forces was verbalized by one of a group of radical medical students in this way: "There is a tension between the traditional deference of the working class toward the upper class, and their sense of conflict with them over many vital aspects of their lives. The place where the classes meet is localized to the medical arena. In other circumstances the classes do not meet." As a result of this cross-pressure, the average working person is not comfortable with the physician. He may not openly challenge the physician's authority, but neither may he comply with the medical recommendations after he gets home.

The historical, cultural, and ideological trends which emerged in the Soviet Union were also critical explanatory variables for physician power, but of quite a different sort. Three factors in particular merit attention: the impact of the death and destruction of World War II, the pervasiveness of medical oversight coupled with citizen obligation to attend to his health, and the special ambience attached to the fact that so many primary care physicians are women.

Although the Second World War severely damaged Britain, its land was not invaded, and the rate of civilian casualties was less than that endured in the U.S.S.R. Accordingly the war is still a very salient issue there, at an intensity difficult for the American visitor to comprehend. Mass graves and monuments to war heroes constantly remind the public of the suffering of the period, when there were 20 million dead. An example of the continued concern is the custom for brides in many cities to place their bridal bouquets on the tomb of the local World War II unknown soldier, immediately after the ceremony. During the war, the physicians were literally life savers, and their role in rescuing and treating victims under bombing and artillery fire is remembered by anyone over 40 today. The possibility of challenging a doctor's decision in such situations of danger and stress undoubtedly did not often arise, while the physicians' self-sacrificing attention to the needs of the injured was evident. Attitudes from that period have clearly carried over to the present. For example, respondents to a survey undertaken by one of the regional polyclinics for its district, showed that some of the physicians received high praise because they were "just like doctors in the war: very concerned, very active, very willing to help."[4]

Another facet of the Soviet medical system difficult for Westerners to understand is the all-pervasiveness of health supervision. Children and students must be examined periodically in the schools, through the special maternal and child health clinics. They receive checkups before being allowed to go to summer camp. As for adults, no one who is working can escape. The need for periodic examinations in order to continue employment has already been alluded to. Tourist guides, because they meet all kinds of foreigners and their germs, are given annual innoculations; some of the young women try to get out of it to no avail; the physician comes to the office to do the job. According to several informants, there are medical stations in every area of major industrial establishments, satellites of the enterprise polyclinic, where physicians and "feldshers" — specially trained intermediate health personnel (Sidel, 1968) — are located. They get to know the workers well, check on their health, follow up those with chronic conditions, lecture on health matters, and monitor compliance with safety and sanitary rules. Women workers are given regular gynecological examinations whether they want them or not. One polyclinic doctor stated that in industry every employee has a "sports rating," and the "coffee break" is an "exercise break," with calisthenics for fifteen minutes. This physician noted that some managed to slip away and have a smoke in the washroom instead. Workers who are recalcitrant and refuse to follow the doctor's treatment recommendations, or insist on treatment for ailments which the doctor considers imaginary, will be put in the hospital as inpatients for a complete workup and specialist's examination.

Moreover the regional polyclinic structure permits close health supervision in the neighborhoods. One physician with long experience in one such polyclinic told the researcher about how well she knew her blocks of families. They called her "Aunt M——," she was invited to weddings and funerals, and made social visits as well as house calls. She felt that if she noticed someone not looking well, she would be able to urge him or her to get a medical examination, because everyone in her district trusted her, they knew her so well. Several polyclinics explained the system of patient follow-up. If someone with a chronic condition, for example, fails to keep a regular checkup appointment he is sent a letter or postcard. If this fails to work a nurse visits him, then visits his family, and as a last resort the manager of the enterprise where he works will be asked to get him to come in.

In this all-encompassing atmosphere, many polyclinic doctors interviewed seemed to find it hard to imagine any serious challenge of a physician's expertise, or to view the admitted examples of questioning physician authority as anything but examples of aberrant behavior. At an enterprise polyclinic, the chief of staff said, "The doctor doesn't tell the worker how to work and does not expect the worker to tell the doctor how to take care of his responsibility." The fact is, however, that patients do perceive differences in physician ability and sources of medical care. Thus one informant suggested that enterprise polyclinics were better than regional ones, because both union and management, as well as the establishment's political committee, were concerned with the quality of the medical care. These clinics were able, with union-negotiated funds, to provide better equipment and pay higher salaries, thus attracting more able staff. According to this informant, regional polyclinics catered largely to pensioners, an opinion not incongruent with research observations. Also there is a small private practice sector chiefly in the form of cooperatives of male specialists, in a few cities and in the South, and some of the intelligentsia prefer these services if they are seriously ill.

Public acceptance of the pervasiveness of the medical system is partly ideological. There is apparently a strong sense that maintaining one's own health is an obligation of citizenship. It is a person's public duty to keep well, and if ill, to get well. In this effort, cooperation with the health practitioners is part of the obligation. Indeed this ideology has been incorporated into law, on both a national and individual republic basis. One polyclinic director displayed copies of the legislation for the Ukrainian Republic, whose preamble states that the attitude of a person to his own health is a concern of the state. Thus in the U.S.S.R. the Parsonian conception of the sick role as including the obligation to get well (Parsons, 1951) has been institutionalized in the formal legal structure.[5]

Perhaps another basis for the acceptance of all-encompassing medical attention is social-psychological, and is related to the fact that most primary care physicians, and indeed most physicians, have been women, a statistic true at least since 1940. The constant oversight, the continued concern about health, the persistent follow-ups and reminders about taking care of oneself are reminiscent of a mothering role. This impression grew during the data collection, as polyclinic after polyclinic was visited, and the researcher was introduced to many women physicians — in medical departments, minor surgery, orthopedics, and all the other sections of the medical center — and often they were indeed maternal in appearance and manner.

One non-medical informant actually verbalized the mother ambience by talking about an instance where he had a false reading of high blood pressure, and had quite an argument with the doctor who wanted him to change his entire life style. The doctor talked to him "like a grandmother about all the dangers of not caring for himself and was shocked at his cavalier attitude."

The evidence is scanty and impressionistic but the hypothesis could be formulated that the acceptance of medical intrusion into so many aspects of Soviet life — work, recreation, education — is related to the fact that mothers are expected to worry about the well-being of their children, even into adulthood. And in many cultures, societal values dictate that at all ages it is a good thing to listen to your mother; as a child you obey; as an adult you at least should try to comply with her wishes. The image of the health-provider as a mother figure is indeed congruent with family health care patterns in many societies, not just in the U.S.S.R.

Implications for the Future of Physician Authority

A first review of the field data has suggested some answers to the queries which initiated this research. Across two quite different societies, individual as well as societal characteristics modify the knowledge-power model of the physician's role. Education of the patient does make a difference in acceptance of physician advice, and in some instances interacts with age to undermine authority. Level of bureaucratization of the medical care delivery systems seems, however, to have less meaning for physician power than the way in which medical workers are used by bureaucratic structures as gatekeepers and enforcers of the system. Although the level of bureaucratization of health care varied between the two social systems, in both cases the practitioner's position was strengthened as a result of his or her control over access to non-medical benefits.

The more salient factors affecting medical practitioners' authority and status were, on the other hand, not included in the original knowledge-power model or reflected in the original research questions. These are the historical, cultural, and ideological variables.[6] Traditional imputations of power based on social-class position, the impact of experiences like a devastating war, and institutionalized beliefs in individual health responsibility, appear to have major consequences for the role and authority of the physician. Finally, the sex of the practitioner may have a social-psychological meaning unlike that originally expected, for being a woman may undergird physician authority rather than diminish it, by invoking a mother image.

Doctors have been viewed as the prototype of the occupational category, profession, approaching on all parameters the ideal-typical end of the continua of professional characteristics. What then are the implications of these findings for the future relation of knowledge and authority among professionals, and particularly physicians?

Consider first the key characteristic of the physician's autonomy, the right granted by society and validated by licensure to define and carry out his tasks. The expression and realization of this autonomy shifts from the *societal* level to that of *individual* transactions with clients at the point of actual task performance. While at this stage physician autonomy is operationalized as authority over patients, theoretically it continues to be grounded in the characteristics of the occupation. The findings here tend to nullify that contention. Degree of authority over clients depends in part on *client* characteristics rather than occupational characteristics alone, i.e., on age and education of the patients. Although these variables affect authority through the instrumentality of patient claims to knowledge conflicting with and undermining physician claims to knowledge monopoly, the fact remains that client characteristics have not heretofore been included in the core model of profession,[7] and have been neglected in the concept of the sick role. Indeed when such characteristics are given weight in studies of compliance with physicians' treatment recommendations, they are viewed as obstacles to obedience rather than source of challenge (McKinlay, 1972).

From another perspective, the critical role of knowledge monopoly is negated by examination of the physician's gatekeeper activities. Professional power is based less on special knowing than on assignment of authority by an organization, and conclusions are reached less on medical than on interactional and bureaucratic grounds. When a doctor is confronted with a worker who has taken a few days off and wants to be paid, the decision to grant the leave has virtually nothing to do with the professional's special expertise. Consideration of his own time pressures at the moment of the request, implications for later requests, the importance of keeping the worker's good will, the possible reactions of the employer, the number of such requests previously granted and their cumulative effect, all enter the decision-making process of the gatekeeper. They equal if not exceed the issue of the actual medical situation of the applicant.

Similarly when a physician becomes a facilitator for housing, phone service, vacations, and the like, he is not as a rule calling up any particular medical expertise. It does not take years of training to recognize that an old lady living alone will need a telephone in the event of an illness emergency. However, the welfare system has been set up to require the physician's validation of a request for this scarce resource, and his power comes from that bureaucratic arrangement rather than from his medical degree.

The variables of history, culture, and ideology are also outside the parameters of the medical model as generally conceptualized. The data on the meaning of traditional class position for compliance with physician authority in Britain reveal that the possession of specialized knowledge is a *post hoc* explanation and justification for a social reality with roots in the past.[8] The findings that medical technology can have differing impacts on physician power depending on cultural setting — in Britain it is said to detract, in the U.S.S.R. to enhance, a doctor's authority — again imply that it is not claims to specialized expertise per se, but societal interpretations of the significance of these claims which are governing.

As for the ideological variable, there have been a few indications in the recent literature that this is an important factor in physicians' status. The ideological content of the "new professional" movement and attendant demands for professional accountability is quite explicit, as are the deprofessionalization exhortations addressed to medicine in the sparse information out of mainland China (Haug, 1973). The validity of this factor is reinforced by the present research, particularly in the data from the U.S.S.R., where the ideology of citizen responsibility for health maintenance and for illness treatment is the rationale for public acquiescence to a pervasive system of medical oversight, and explains the formal obligation to accede to physician advice. Although not necessarily incongruent with the theory of profession which distinguishes certain occupations as having special knowledge, humanitarian concerns and derivative autonomy, it adds a new dimension to the theory, redefining the circumstances under which the core characteristics provide a meaningful definition of the concept.

It is possible to summarize these findings and their theoretical implications by stating that data from both Great Britain and the U.S.S.R. confirm the American-based impression that professional authority is eroding, at least in part as a result of client education, and that the medical profession is no exception to this development, although the pace of change varies in different societies. Perhaps more important, it can be said that the model of profession and of medicine based on occupational characteristics is at best incomplete and at worst erroneous. Factors such as client characteristics, societal structure, and ideology may match if not outweigh the occupational parameters.

The hypothesis takes shape that the segments of the division of labor currently entitled "profession" in the West are simply a range of occupations which require greater or lesser degrees of training and expertise, and in which clients, also with greater or lesser knowledge of the tasks that occupation performs, negotiate a course of action designed to accomplish some individually or socially desirable end. Factors affecting this negotiation are the bureaucratic structures in which the transactions occur, the ideological themes which place values on different transactional styles and outcomes, and the historical events and traditions which in various social and cultural settings have patterned practitioner and client beliefs and behaviors. The underlying model is one of expert and consumer, without the moral and evaluative overtones of the professional model. While the data presented here cannot support this hypothesis, they at least suggest the theoretical utility of systematic exploration of its validity.

FOOTNOTES

1. It might be argued that the voluminous literature on failures and factors in patient compliance (Marston, 1970; McKinlay, 1972) indicate that not following a physician's advice is a common phenomenon. Although this is undoubtedly the case (Freidson, 1961), compliance and non-compliance as such are not logically equivalent to acceptance-rejection of physician authority. Patients can accept medical authority, that is the right to advise and the obligation to obey, but still fail to fulfill that obligation by complying. Conversely, in terms of the bargaining-negotiating

model of the medical encounter (Balint, 1957), it is possible that a patient complies with a regimen because he has bent the practitioner to his will, securing the diagnosis and treatment plan which he was desirous of having confirmed when entering the interaction.

2. Quotation marks represent statements reconstructed from notes and tapes, not always exact quotes, particularly in the U.S.S.R., where respondents were translated.

3. Personal communication from Martin Bridgestock, Medical Sociology Research Centre, Swansea, Wales.

4. As an aside, the survey showed that complaints of the patients in the U.S.S.R. echoed those reported in the United Kingdom (Klein, 1972): lack of attentiveness, rudeness, hasty care. In both countries even these complaints were rare.

5. For a further discussion of the Soviet health system, with a similar perspective, see James E. Muller et al. (1972).

6. For a more detailed discussion of these issues with reference to Great Britain, see Haug (1976).

7. One exception to this generalization is the work of Terence Johnson (1972). In *Professions and Power* he suggests that in the case of corporate clients, authority may flow from a client to professional instead of vice versa. Unfortunately, this monograph is little known in the United States, and not too easy to secure.

8. Krause (1971:111), one of the few occupational sociologists to include the historical perspective, makes a similar point concerning the medical profession.

BIBLIOGRAPHY

Balint, Michael
1957   The Doctor, His Patient and the Illness. New York: International Universities Press, Inc.

Becker, Howard S.
1962   "The nature of a profession." Pp. 27-46 in Education for the Professions, Sixty-first Yearbook of the National Society for the Study of Education, Part II. Chicago: The University of Chicago Press.

Boston Women's Health Book Collective
1973   Our Bodies Our Selves. New York: Simon and Schuster.

Eulau, Heinz
1973   "Skill revolution and consultative commonwealth." American Political Science Review 62 (March): 169-191.

Freidson, Eliot
1961   Patients' Views of Medical Practice. New York: Russell Sage Foundation.
1970   Professional Dominance. New York: Atherton Press, Inc.

Geiger, H. Jack
1972   "The new doctor." In Gross, Ronald, and Paul Osterman
        (eds.), The New Professions. New York: Simon and Schuster.

Goode, William J.
1969   "The theoretical limits of professionalization." Pp. 266-313
        in Etzioni, Amitai (ed.), The Semi-Professions and Their
        Organizations. New York: The Free Press.

Haug, Marie R.
1973   "Deprofessionalization — an alternative hypothesis for the
        future." The Sociological Review Monograph No. 20
        (December): 195-211.
1974   "Computer technology and the obsolescence of the concept of
        profession." Paper presented at the 8th World Congress of
        Sociology, Toronto (Canada) August (Session II of the Research
        Committee on Work).
1975   "The deprofessionalization of everyone." Sociological Focus 8
        (August): 197-214.
1976   "Issues in general practitioner authority in the National
        Health Service." In Stacey, Margaret (ed.), The Sociology of
        the National Health Service. Monograph of the (British)
        Sociological Review.

Haug, Marie R. and Marvin B. Sussman
1969   "Professional autonomy and the revolt of the client." Social
        Problems 17 (Fall): 153-161.

Johnson, Terence J.
1972   Professions and Power. London: The Macmillan Press Ltd.

Klein, Rudolf
1972   Complaints Against Doctors. London: Charles Knight &
        Co. Ltd.

Krause, Elliott A.
1971   The Sociology of Occupations. Boston: Little, Brown and
        Company.

Lefkowitz, Annie, and Marlene Ausmus
1970   "Opportunities in subprofessional health occupations."
        Occupational Outlook Quarterly 14 (Winter): 6-18.

Marston, M.
1970   "Compliance with medical regimens: a review of the literature."
        Nursing Research 19 (July-August): 312-323.

McKinlay, John B.
1972   "Some approaches and problems in the study of the use of
        services — an overview." Journal of Health and Social
        Behavior 13 (June): 115-152.

Mechanic, David
1970   "Correlates of frustration among British general practitioners."
Journal of Health and Social Behavior 11 (June): 87-104.

Moore, Wilbert E.
1970   The Professions: Roles and Rules. New York: Russell Sage
Foundation.

Muller, James E., Faye G. Abdellah, F.T. Billings, Arthur E. Hess, Donald Petit, and Rober O. Egeberg
1972   "The Soviet health system — aspects of relevance for
medicine in the United States." New England Journal of
Medicine 286 (March 30): 693-702.

Parsons, Talcott
1951   The Social System. New York: The Free Press.

Perrow, Charles
1972   Complex Organizations, A Critical Essay. Glenview, Illinois:
Scott Foresman and Company.

Reeder, Leo G.
1972   "The patient-client as consumer: some observations on the
changing professional client relationship." Journal of Health
and Human Behavior 13 (December): 406-412.

Reiff, Robert
1971   "The danger of the techni-pro: democratizing the human
service professions." Social Policy 2 (May-June): 62-64.

Schwartz, W.B.
1970   "Medicine and the computer: the promise and problems of
change." New England Journal of Medicine 283 (December 3):
1257-1264.

Sidel, Victor
1968   "Feldshers and feldsherism I and II." New England Journal
of Medicine 278 (April 25): 934-939, and (May 2): 987-992.

U.S. Bureau of the Census
1972   Statistical Abstract of the United States. 93rd edition.
Washington, D.C.

Wilensky, Harold
1964   "The professionalization of everyone?" American Journal
of Sociology 70 (September): 137-158.

The Care of the Patient

Introduction

The importance of understanding illness behaviour, patients' self-concept and other sociological, psychological and cultural aspects of patient care is presented in this section. The impact of illness on the person is by far the most important knowledge to understand because the uniqueness of this human experience is at the very heart of our humanistic thinking. It is to this state — the psycho-social concomitants of the illness experience — that we now turn.

The ethical mandate which flows from this understanding should not result in anything but a humanistic approach in our field. Cultural and social factors, religious beliefs, psychological climate and sociological forces all have a profound effect on the experience of illness and must be carefully considered if the humanistic concept is to have a meaningful relation to reality. If we chose to ignore the psycho-social aspects of illness, it is at the peril of our patients; and our own peril as professionals and individuals.

This section begins with a selection by Daisy Tagliacozzo and Hans O. Mauksch; "The Patient's View of the Patient's Role." In an extensive and incisive study, Tagliacozzo and Mauksch contribute a significant dimension to understanding how patients view their roles in a large metropolitan hospital. Their discussion is based "on a study which sought to ascertain to what extent the attitudes and needs which are organized around these two experiences, being ill and being hospitalized, may differ or even come into conflict with each other."

A study which investigates the attitudes and behaviour of surgical patients and the reactions of doctors and nurses to that behaviour, is presented in the second article "Good Patients and Problem Patients: Conformity and Deviance in a General Hospital" by Judith Lorber. Previous research had suggested that medical personnel encourage trust, cooperation, uncomplainingness, and undemandingness in patients, but that not all patients subscribe to these norms to the same degree. This study found that patients did differ in the extent of their acceptance of "good - patient" norms, and, as predicted, that those who did not completely accept them were less submissive to hospital routines than were patients who did completely accept them. The doctors and nurses interrupted well-established routines and made extra work for their "problem patients," but how such patients were treated depended on the severity of their illness. Possible consequences of being labelled a problem patient are: premature discharge, neglect, and referral to a psychiatrist.

In "Gaining Awareness of Cultural Difference: A Case Example" Raphella Sohier emphasizes the importance of the health practitioner having an understanding of cultural factors in patient care. Sohier illustrates this principle from her experience as a nurse in the Jewish community in Antwerp, Belgium. "Total care," she concludes "can become a reality only when patients are seen in the framework of their individual cultural patterns."

The importance of maintaining and protecting the dignity of patients when they are ill is analyzed in our fourth selection, "Illness and Indignity" by Thomas S. Szasz. He points out that "it is not enough that we do a technically competent job of healing the patient's body; we must do an equally competent job of safeguarding his dignity and self-esteem."

This section is completed with a contribution by Leo G. Reeder; "The Patient - Client as a Consumer: Some Observations on the Changing Professional - Client Relationship." Professional - client relations are considered in the context of certain structural changes in society, especially in the health-care field. These societal features are discussed in terms of development of consumerism as a force for changing the professional - client relationship, particularly in bureaucratic settings.

The Patient's View of the Patient's Role

Daisy L. Tagliacozzo and Hans O. Mauksch

Every society grants to the sick person special privileges and every society also imposes on the sick person certain obligations.[1] An understanding of such general norms can provide an effective guide to the study of the behavior and attitudes of the sick in our society. However, general norms gain meaning in a specific social setting, or may be modified by intra-institutional expectations. The extent to which a sick person may feel free to seek satisfaction for his emotional needs and to assume the "rights and privileges of the sick role" may thus depend on the social context within which behavior unfolds. Even if general rules for behavior remain the same, the patient may be influenced by considerations which involve efforts to accommodate to real or imagined expectations of significant others.

The experience of being hospitalized adds another dimension to the experience of being ill. This dimension consists of the rights and obligations which are legitimated by organizational forces and which are based on the fact that admission to the hospital is tantamount to assuming an organizational position with all the implications for normative compliance and sanctions. This discussion is based on a study which sought to ascertain to what extent the attitudes and needs which are organized around these two experiences, being ill and being hospitalized, may differ or even come into conflict with each other. The attitudes and reactions of patients were viewed within the context of a system of roles and as a consequence of the patient's efforts to conform to perceived systems of expectations. The study concentrated on the implications of hospitalization, with less concern for the illness role *per se*. It explored to what extent the role of the hospitalized patient may be lacking clear definitions of rights and easily definable criteria for legitimate claims. The question was raised whether the position and the attitudes of patients deprive them of genuine means to control others in the system and thus limit their readiness to express their claims and desires without fear of sanction.

Throughout the study the patient is shown to be aware of the degree to which he is dependent on those who care for him. This dependency is

From *Patients, Physicians and Illness*, edited by E.G. Jaco, Macmillan Publishing Co. Inc., 1972. By permission of the authors.
Based on a study conducted by the authors through the Department of Patient Care Research, Presbyterian St. Luke's Hospital, Chicago, Ill. This study was supported by a grant from the Commonwealth Fund.

based largely on the power to heal and to cure. It is also based on the power ascribed to hospital functionaries to give or to withhold those daily services which, for the hospitalized patient, can embrace some basic survival needs. The single or double rooms and the rapid patient turnover in the modern hospital do not foster an effective patient community which could serve as interpreter and modifier of hospital rules. The patient, therefore, is much more dependent on his previous learning, be it from direct or indirect experiences with the patient role. More importantly, the absence of adequate interpretations by the patient community makes the patient more dependent on hospital functionaries for clues about the appropriateness of his behavior, demands and expectations.

The fact that patients frequently remain strangers in the hospital community tends to add to the power of those who, as functionaries, are intimately familiar with the rules and expectations of the organization. The power which is vested in them can inhibit the patient to seek clarification and guidance. Also, those who are informed tend to become oblivious to the needs of their clients to be initiated into the "rules of the game."

The study was conducted in a metropolitan voluntary hospital with a capacity of 850 beds. The hospital is part of a large Midwest medical center. It is a teaching hospital for nurses and physicians. Patients occupy predominantly two-bed or private rooms.[2] This discussion rests on the analysis of 132 interviews which were administered to 86 patients. The sample was limited to patients who were admitted with cardiovascular or gastro-intestinal diagnoses. All patients in the sample were Caucasian, American-born males or females between 40 and 60 years of age. All patients had been previously hospitalized and all were married. They paid for their hospitalization in part with private or industrial insurance. During the semi-structured interview, the patient was asked to express himself freely on present and previous hospital experiences. The interviews averaged one hour and were recorded and transcribed. The average day of interviewing was the fifth day of hospitalization. When possible, second interviews were conducted.

Physicians and Nurses: Their Significance

Physicians and nurses are among the significant others in the network of role relationships in which the hospitalized patient becomes involved. Their significance is derived from different sources. The physician represents authority and prestige. His orders legitimize the patient's demands on others and justify otherwise deviant aspects of illness behavior. The physician is not only the "court of appeal" for exemption from normal role responsibilities,[3] he also functions as the major legitimizing agent for the patient's demands during hospitalization. Yet his orders generally do not constitute guides to behavior in specific situations and they do not consider or modify the patient's understanding of the formal and informal expectations of nurses. Although the physician's authority ranks supreme in the eyes of most patients, they are also aware that he is only intermittently present and thus not in a position to evaluate the behavior of both patients and nurses and to sanction this behavior during the everyday procedures of hospital care.

The significance of the nurse stems not only from her authority in interpreting, applying and enforcing the orders of the physician but, in addition, from the fact that she can judge and react to the patient's behavior more continuously than the physician. From the patient's point of view, he also depends upon the nurse as an intermediary in the provision of many other institutional services.

For most patients it is of greatest importance to feel that they adjust to the expectations of the nurse and of the physician. To accommodate themselves to what they feel is expected of them, patients must be able to perceive these expectations as congruent or they must cope with the strains involved in efforts to adjust to what may appear to them as conflicting demands. Conflict is thus likely to arise if the nurse executes a plan of care which, from the point of view of the patient, deviates in detail or emphasis from the patient's interpretation of the physician's orders.

Close adherence to the orders of the physician was not equally important for all patients and not all patients appear to be equally intense in their sensitivity to congruence in the plan of care and cure. Those patients who expressed concern for complete adherence to the physician's word and expected strictest observance and literal interpretation of medical orders typically expressed distrust in the reliability and efficiency of anyone except the physician. These patients frequently feared that even minor deviations may result in further physical harm. For some patients, close adherence to medical orders appeared congruent with their conceptions of themselves; as did some patients, who resisted following certain medical orders, they used this area of conformity to convey something essential about themselves.

Demands for rigid adherence to medical orders were associated with the desire for "reliable" nursing care and "efficiency." The eagerly co-operative patient not only emphasized that he followed all orders willingly, he also expected the nurse to "co-operate" with him in his efforts to carry out the orders of the physician as he understood them. The patient's concern typically expressed itself in close observations of hospital personnel, in emphasis on observance of punctuality and in worry whether "orders have been written" and "charts double-checked." Such efforts to "co-operate with the physician" by seeing that "things get done" may become a source of stress. The patient who is ready to act on behalf of medical orders may have to call for services from the nurse and impose demands on her time or ask her to alter behavior. Thus, if the patient hears from the physician that the "specimen should be warm," he may feel obligated to insist that a "cooling-off" delay be avoided. If the physician has told him that he may "stay in bed another day," the patient's interpretation may lead him to actively resist a nurse's urging that he do some things for himself: "My doctor said that I can stay in bed another day." Patients' insistence on rigid adherence to the orders of the physician were frequently defended in the light of one implication of the sick role — the obligation to make efforts towards the restoration of health. Thus, patients who were critical of deviations from medical orders justified their criticisms by pointing out that they did not want to be "complainers" or "troublemakers" — but that they, after all, "want to get well."

When a patients's efforts to co-operate fully and to observe the details of medical orders expressed themselves in more frequent demands, he also reacted to the risks involved in violating his obligation not to be demanding of nurses. Those patients who reported that they had expressed their desire for compliance with medical orders in active demands or complaints also tended to be very observant of the reactions of members of the nursing staff. Praise and criticism of "good" and "bad" nurses revealed that these patients rejected the nurse who "grumbled" and that they praised enthusiastically the nurse who responded "willingly" and who "smiled" when she was asked to do things for the patient. Patients also praised the nurse who "helped the patient to co-operate" and who "did not mind" when she was reminded of an order.

Those patients for whom co-operation with a physician's order became the guiding principle during hospitalization tended to be very sensitized to the reactions of others. They appeared to be "on the alert" and reacted quickly to facial expression, a tone of voice and the general manner in which a request was received. If they felt that their demands were not well received, they frequently became angered and, when given an opportunity, expressed their antagonism in attacks on those members of the nursing staff who "do not treat you like a person," who "make you feel that you are at their mercy" and "who consider you just a case."

The conflict between the felt obligation to insist on precise implementation of medical orders and efforts not to appear demanding or inconsiderate vis à vis the nursing staff was often resolved in favor of striving for approval by nurses. The data indicate that many patients prefer not to risk appearing too demanding or too dependent. They accept what appears to them to be deviations from the physician's orders, and even violate what they believe is expected of them by the physician. They anxiously watch a medication being late , rather than object to the delay, and they watch the specimen get cold rather than pointing this out to a nurse. Frequently this endeavor to "please" the nurse may backfire. Patients who disobey the physician's orders and get up to do "small things" for themselves rather than call the nurse may find themselves reprimanded by her because she may view this as lack of co-operation or even protest. She also may consider such behavior an incident which could incur the anger of the physician.

Thus, patients may pay for the security of "being liked" by nurses and of having them "know that I am not demanding" with concerns over arousing the physician's criticism or harming their own recovery. But even where the obligation to be cooperative with the physician is not immediately at stake, patients may somewhat reluctantly forego the privileges which they could claim as a result of being sick. As one patient expressed it:

> If it is a hotel you won't hesitate to pick up a phone or to complain; in a hospital you think twice about it — you figure maybe they are busy or shorthanded.... It's a much more human thing, the hospital. . . it's more personal.

Expectations and Constraints

When patients were asked what was expected of them by their physicians and by nurses, they responded with considerable consistency, indicating that several rules for "proper" conduct of patients were well defined and widely shared. The physician was seen as expecting "co-operation" and "trust and confidence." A large group of patients felt that the nurse, too, expected "co-operation." On the other hand, many patients were convinced that nurses expected them "not to be demanding," to be "respectful" and to be "considerate." Only very few patients listed these latter three categories for physicians.

Self-descriptions which patients introjected into the interviews followed a similar pattern. It was most important to patients that the interviewer saw them as having "trust and confidence" in those who took care of them. This was particularly true of those patients who also admitted to some negative reactions toward nurses or physicians. Many patients were eager to mention that they were not demanding, co-operative, not dependent and considerate. In spontaneous discussions of the obligations of the hospitalized patient, the pattern did not change significantly.

One of the factors underlying the patient's hesitation to impose demands on hospital personnel is his awareness of the presence of other, often sicker patients. Observation of other patients introduces restraints. Comparisons of "my illness" with the illness of the roommate appeared to intensify the moral obligation to "leave them free to take care of the seriously ill" and comparisons of one's own claims or criticisms with the behavior of a very ill person seemed to intensify restrained behavior: "After I observed him I felt kind of bad. I felt that I should be grateful and not ask for anything." It is well nigh impossible and a latent source of difficulty for the patient to judge his comparative status relative to patients in other rooms. The nurse summoned to give him a glass of water may have been called away from "a critical case." The isolation of the patient and the ensuing inability to establish relative claims serve as restraining forces on the expression of needs,[4] even though this concern is counterbalanced with an occasionally voiced concern about "getting one's share."

The patient's perceived entitlement for service is also linked to his definition of the severity of his illness. Patients apparently feel more secure in ascertaining their rights if their understanding of their condition permits them to rank themselves in the upper strata of a "hierarchy of illness." However, a secure assessment of "my case" may be difficult. Communications from the physician are general and understanding of the relative severity of the illness does not appear to be facilitated by his explanations. In many cases, a statement such as "I want you to stay in bed" does not legitimize the demand for a glass of water — the patient gets up to avoid being considered "too demanding."

Patients therefore seem to link the extent of their claims on service to readily perceived and objectively visible indices. Thus, being in traction, having tubes attached or being restrained by dressings are highly ranked legitimators for patients' demands. Fever also serves as a criterion for claims; the patient who asks the nurse what his temperature might be not only may inquire about the severity of his illness but indirectly may also ask: "To what services am I entitled today?" Hospital rules which prevent the nurse from giving such information may deny the patient guidelines for the rules applicable to his behavior.

Two-thirds of all patients in the sample indicated that they had refrained from expressing their needs and criticisms at least once. The observation that nurses are too busy, rushed and overworked was given as the most frequent reason for this reluctance. Beliefs about the conditions under which hospital personnel work serve thus as another limiting factor in the patient's expression of demands. One has to keep in mind the admiration for nurses and for "all those who do such difficult work" to understand why some patients may spend a night helping another patient when being told "that there is a shortage on the nightshift." Some patients did not engage in these activities without some conflict. They admitted that they were concerned with the physician's reactions "if he finds out," and that they were fearful of the consequences of such activity for their health. Even though they never admitted it directly, many responses revealed indirectly their desire to take more advantage of the privileges of the sick.

Constraint in voicing demands was also reinforced by the patient's assessment of the power of hospital personnel and physicians relative to his own. Over one-fourth of those patients who admitted to restraint of their demands also expressed their often resentful assessment of their own helplessness. Efforts to be "considerate" of the conditions which limit services may thus be convenient rationalizations of the patient's fears of offending others and of endangering his good relationship with them. "Being on good terms" was seen by these patients not only as a convenient but as an essential factor for their welfare. They directly expressed their awareness of their inability to control those who are in charge of their care. Patients felt that they were subject to rewards and punishment and that essential services can be withheld unless they make themselves acceptable. Some of these patients were dependent upon intimate forms of physical assistance, and their points of view reflected their awareness of this dependence upon others.

Feelings of helplessness were directly expressed in observations that "one is at their mercy," that "trying to change things is futile" and "won't get you anywhere" and that patients feel "helpless." The recognition of the power of others to withhold services also found expression in fears that one does not want to be considered a "complainer," or "trouble-maker" or a "demanding patient," and in such apprehensions as "they can refuse to answer your bell, you know," or "they can refuse to make your bed." The same fears were expressed in efforts "to save that button so they come when I really need them" or in enthusiastic reactions to nurses who "come in to inquire why you never call for them" or who "do not mind if you ring once too often."

Patients very rarely expressed openly a concern that their physician may impose sanctions on inappropriate behavior. They tried to be intensely considerate toward him, since he, too, is considered "very busy" and "on his way" to other sick patients. Attempts to accommodate demands to these pressures on the physician serve as a considerable restraint on the patient's willingness to ask questions.

The admiration for the physician was in most cases tied to a very personal and emotionally charged attachment to the man who is "so kind and understanding." Gratitude intensified efforts to "make things easy" for him. Although hostility or annoyances toward nurses was often directly expressed, patients actively resisted direct verbalization of any negative feelings toward "the physician." Typically, complaints were expressed reluctantly and in terms of "I wish he could" coupled with quick modifications such as "I know he can't — he is too busy."

Patients may also be concretely limited by the observation that the physician is "on the go." Thus, a patient may want to ask questions and feel that "taking his time" is legitimate, but may feel that the time is simply not made available:

He'll say well, we'll talk about it next time. And next time he'll talk fast, he out-talks you — and rushes out of the room and then when he's out of the room you think, well, I was supposed to ask him what he's going to do about my medicine . . . you run in the hall and he has disappeared that fast.

A patient who was impressed with the fact that his physician was "over-burdened and rushed" tried to describe how the resulting pressure of his own tensions and anxiety prevented him from fully comprehending what he was told:

All I know is that your mind sort of runs ahead. You sort of anticipate what they are going to say, and you finish what they are going to say in your mind. I guess it's because perhaps sometimes you have trouble following them or maybe you would want them to say certain things, and you are listening — well, I don't know . . . you try to think what they are going to say, because otherwise, you have difficulty understanding them, but then, when they are out of the room, you don't remember a thing about what they have said.

In view of the above, it is not surprising that patients who were asked directly what they "considered their rights" had some difficulties responding. One-fourth of the respondents admitted that they did not know what their rights were; some patients stated outright that they had no rights. The majority of respondents limited themselves to general answers such as "good care," followed by the modification that specific claims depended upon the "seriousness of the illness." The belief that claims for service had to be justified in terms of immediate physical needs over-shadowed any inclination to voice the rights of paying consumers. Few patients justified their demands in relation to their monetary payment and many of those who introduced the criteria of a paying consumer quickly added to their demands other legitimizing factors, such as the nature of their illness or the fact that they had been considerate in other respects. Conceptions of rights and obligations provide guidelines for alternative actions. They are used and "fitted" in accordance with the exigencies of situations and the developing meanings which individuals and groups bring to bear upon them. The general patterns which have been discussed should not conceal that differences in the characteristics of patients may contribute to significant variations in the more general theme. The following observations will illustrate the importance of further research in this area.

Patients who do not experience active and well-defined symptoms and whose activities are not visibly impaired may hesitate to present themselves to others as seriously ill and may find "co-operation" at times more difficult. Patients with cardio-vascular illness tended to focus more frequently on behavior involving co-operation with physicians and nurses; particularly in relation to the physician, this obligation appeared to preoccupy these patients. They were also more intent on presenting themselves as co-operative to the interviewer. Some of these patients were severely ill from the medical point of view, requiring complete bed rest and its concomitant extensive services. However, they seemed to have a difficult time accepting this state without concern that they may be considered "too dependent" or overly "demanding." At times, these difficulties appeared enhanced by social and economic pressures to leave the hospital, and by psychological needs for denial which also seemed to find expression in the insistence that they "really did not need any special attention" and that they were "not worried about their illness."

Some of the subtle difficulties of these patients are not easily verbalized. Only rarely can a patient formulate as forcefully the aftermath of a heart attack as did the patient quoted below. His statement sums up the illusions and hints dropped by other patients with a cardiac problem:

> Well, you know, a heart patient is a peculiar animal. That heart attack has done something to him, not only physically but mentally. I can tell you this because I have been through it. It brings up something which you don't want to let go of. If he tells you you must stay in bed, well, how come this sudden change? I don't want to stay in bed, and if he tells you that you cannot walk upstairs, he is telling you that you are weak, that you are no longer strong. He has taken something away from you — ah, your pride. You suddenly want to do what you are not supposed to do, what you have been doing all your life and that you have every right to do. Besides, a heart patient has an excitability built up in him.

Patients with cardio-vascular conditions verbalized criticisms less frequently than other patients. On the other hand, they stressed the importance of "dedication and interest" when discussing their ideal expectations of nurses and physicians.

One explanation for these tendencies may be found in some common fears which occur among patients who suffer from a type of illness in which the onset of a crisis can be sudden and unpredictable. For a patient with a cardio-vascular illness, as probably for all patients who fear a sudden turn for the worse, it is of utmost importance to know that someone will be there when the patient really needs help. The need for this type of security is revealed in the following responses of cardio-vascular patients:

I think that there should be somebody out in front there all the time. I think the hospital would back me up on that. . . . . If the patient was really ill, rang the buzzer and nobody was there to get it — no telling what would happen.

Well, as I said, some patients may need more care because they have a more serious illness and when you have a heart disease then you need to be watched much more, also you are more frightened and it is important that somebody is around to watch your pulse.

Patients with non-specific gastro-intestinal conditions were more likely to be preoccupied with cancer. At times this was accompanied by the suspicion that the physician "really knows but will not tell me." Such apprehensions seemed to make it more difficult for the patient to sustain trust and confidence in personnel, particularly the physician.

Openly anxious and critical patients were found more frequently within the gastro-intestinal category. While patients with cardio-vascular conditions appeared to focus attention on concrete services which assured their safety, gastro-intestinal patients seemed more inclined to focus on the qualitative nature of their interactions with nurses and physicians. They were more easily threatened by the attitudes of others, more responsive to "personalized care" and more openly critical when these areas of expectations were not satisfied.

In each culture there is the recognition that it is legitimate to deviate from normal behavior under certain extreme conditions. For these conditions most societies develop differential standards for men and women. In our society men and women are generally not expected to respond in an identical fashion to pain nor are they expected to react identically to illness. We expect that expressive behavior (complaining or moaning) should be more controlled by men, and we frown less when women appear to exploit the illness role through passive and dependent behavior. All patients generally agreed that it was more difficult for men to be patients.

The data indicate that the sex of a patient may substantially affect orientations, needs and reactions to physicians and nurses. Evidence for such differences can be found in many areas. Women were considerably more critical of nursing care than were men, and more frequently expressed fear of negative sanctions from nurses. Women, more than men, emphasized personalized relationships when they discussed the needs of patients. Women were less concerned with problems of co-operation. On the other hand, they tended to focus on nurses' expectations for consideration and respect. When describing their expectations of nurses or when evaluating them, women focused more on personality attributes than men and also gave more emphasis to efficient and prompt care. Women were more critical when a quick response was not forthcoming and they were generally more concerned with efficiency. It is compatible with the male role to receive care and to have someone else maintain the physical surroundings. Women, however, are typically the managers of the home and the performers of major housekeeping tasks. They "know" from experience the standards of personal care and housekeeping, and thus tend to apply them to their judgment of the nursing team. The female patient's concern that the nurse may be critical of her may be indirectly an expression of her awareness that she tends to be demanding.

The more intense emphasis of women on "personality" and "personalized care" may also stem from a relationship which tends to be less personal and less informal than the relationship between nurses and male patients. Unlike his female counterpart, the male patient is probably not too critical of the technical aspect of those functions of the nurse which are reminiscent of the homemaker and mother. He may also derive satisfaction from his relationship to a member of the opposite sex. All this may not only contribute to tolerance of nursing care in general but may give the appearance of more "personalized" relationships. These conjectures may also help to explain the well-known preference nurses have for male patients.

Fears and Apprehensions

Apprehensions and fears are the frequent companions of illness. The nature of the patient's concern springs, on the one hand, from his intense preoccupations with himself, with *his* body and with *his* state of mind. His dependence on others, on the other hand, prompts simultaneous concern with the meaning and consequences of their activities. Once the patient enters the hospital his attention may shift back and forth from himself to others. He is sensitive to any physical changes and watchful of any new and unexplained symptoms. He wonders about the outcome of an examination and about the effectiveness of his treatment. He ponders the reliability of those who are responsible for the many procedures and activities which to the patient remain unknown or unknowable, albeit essential.

Patients are preoccupied with safety in the hospital. This is revealed in the preoccupation with protection from mistakes and neglect which prevails when patients talk about their own needs or the needs of other patients. It is expressed in the nature of their recall of past experiences. Not only do patients concentrate on negative experiences, but they select those occurrences which signify the dangers of neglect and lack of attention. Although patients generally deny that they, themselves, are fearful, they have a tendency to ascribe such feelings to other patients.

These apprehensions cannot be entirely alleviated by admiration for the professional groups who are responsible for his treatment, or by a very favorable relationship to the personal physician. Realistic awareness of the complexity of large organizations or simply the fact that among many competent and interested doctors and nurses there may always be a "few who are not competent" may at least put the patient on the alert. In the words of a male patient with gastro-intestinal illness this fear is expressed as follows:

> When you are really sick, you are at the mercy of the hospital staff. In my opinion, you've got to have luck on your side. You've got to be lucky enough to get key people in the hospital who are really alert and who wish to do a job; and have someone on the shift at the time you need them who want to give the service or you are just out of luck. I think you could die in one of these hospitals of a heart attack before anybody came in to help you.

Perceptions of the patient role make it unlikely that such fears will be openly expressed by many patients. It is one of the obligations of a patient to have "trust and confidence" in those who care for him. The expression of these concerns could thus be interpreted as a failure to conform to these obligations. Also a free expression of concerns is inhibited by the belief that the courageous, sick persons rather than "sissies" are valued and rewarded.

Apprehensions of certain "dangers" may be directly derived from previous experiences which were, to the patient, indicative of lack of competence, neglect, or lack of interest. They also may be derived indirectly from certain widely held conceptions about the nature of "some" doctors and nurses and the conditions under which they work. Thus, the belief that some nurses do not like "demanding patients" leads to the concern of many patients that asking for too much may result in a slow response to a call or in reduced attention to their needs. The belief that some nurses and some physicians may be prone to oversights because they are inevitably overworked and rushed may further contribute to insecurity. Some patients observed with concern that physicians occasionally are "too busy" to spend enough time to listen to their patients or that a nurse "under the pressure of work" may overlook a physician's order or fail to carry it out in time.

There is evidence in the data that both physicians and nurses, in effect, continuously have to prove themselves. Beliefs such as "some doctors are only interested in money," "some doctors are not interested in their patients," "some doctors are hard-hearted," appear as conceptions about "possibilities" which the patient is ready to have dispelled or confirmed upon first contact with a nurse or a physician in the hospital. Negative conceptions about physicians and nurses, therefore, are typically limited to specific individuals. Without this "specificity" in orientation, patients would find it difficult to sustain the trust and confidence which they consider so important.

The patient's search for safety and security in the hospital may also be indirectly expressed in expectations of good physicians and good nurses.

Their behavior or attitudes are seen by the patient as being instrumental in recovery and recuperation. The attitudes of others in the hospital function as clues which are symbolic of good care. From the patient's point of view, the "dedicated nurse" or the nurse who gives "spontaneous and willing services" is a reliable nurse; the "kind" physician who visits the patient regularly is "trustworthy" and "thorough." Mistakes and neglect are more obviously avoided if the nurse responds promptly, if the physician "knows what is going on" and if the nurse is informed about the doctor's intent. A "prompt response" from a nurse appears as one of the most significant indices for establishing trust and confidence in nursing care.

Patients' perspectives are also shaped by the nature of the social process into which they have entered and by the nature of the interactions to which they are exposed. Those patients who were very responsive to the more impersonal phases of patient-care also tended to be among the more apprehensive. Such patients often felt that they were functioning in a situation in which they could not establish effective and meaningful relationships with others. Feelings of "unrelatedness" were expressed directly in the observation that other patients are often "lonely" and "fearful" or that one sometimes feels like "just a case":

> You're no more . . . no more a patient but just a number . . . you dare not ask a question; you know, they're too busy. And they come around, fine, that's it, "we'll see you next time" and that's it. . . .

The very isolation he fears may be aggravated by the patient himself. In his efforts to be "considerate" and "not demanding" he may intensify the consequences of the anonymity and segmentalization he observes in the modern hospital. Efforts to be a "good patient" may, therefore, trigger disappointments and criticisms of those who do not provide services "spontaneously." The demand for "spontaneous services" appears also to stem from the desire to obtain all necessary services and attentions without having to initiate action. Spontaneous services curtail those interactions in which the patient may be viewed as "too demanding" or "difficult."

The interviews suggest that conformity to the patient role may lead to discrepancies between the behavior and the emotional condition of a patient. The calm appearance of the "good patient" may often hide anxieties and tensions which may not come to the attention of physicians or nurses unless relationships develop which do not trigger fear of criticism or sanction. When patients fail to exercise the restraints on behavior which they think appropriate, guilt or fear may be the consequence. Deviation from the good patient model can be threatening to a patient, unless he is convinced that his behavior was, in the eyes of others, legitimate and/or justified by the condition of his illness:

> I know myself that I talked very rudely to my doctor on one occasion. Afterwards I was ashamed of myself. I was sick or I would never act that way. He is kind and understanding. When I apologized, he acted as if nothing happened. He didn't walk out of the room or tell me off or any of the things that I might do after someone talked to me that way. But I know they have to have a lot of patience with us.

Patients practice an economy of demands, based on their own "principles of exchange." They will indeed curtail their less urgent demands to assure for themselves a prompt response during times when they "really need it." Some patients appear to consider themselves entitled to a certain finite quantity of services which they use sparingly to draw upon during periods of crisis, and many patients seem to feel that their entitlement to service is more severely cut by a demand which does not meet the approval of doctors and nurses:

> I says, "I'm saving that button," I says, "When I push that thing you'll know I need help." She smiled . . . they kind of appreciate that. And from that day, all the times I've been in the hospital I have never pushed the button unless it was something that I actually needed . . . not like some people that drive these nurses crazy; pushing it to raise the bed up; five minutes later push it again. "Oh that's a little too high." To me it paid dividends, because every time I pushed that button I got service, every dog-gone time.

Discussion

The hospitalized patient is a "captive" who cannot leave the hospital without serious consequence to himself. These consequences do not only apply to the patient's physical condition. Our society expects efforts of the sick to do everything in their power to get well as soon as possible. Open rebellion against the care by competent professional personnel is, therefore, subject to severe criticism. The obligation to be a "co-operative patient" is learned early in life and, as has been indicated, apparently taken very seriously by most patients. More aggressive interpretations of the patient role are not easily verbalized and, apparently, not often realistic alternatives for the patient. Prevalent images of the hospital as a crisis institution, the conception that rights and demands should be governed by the seriousness of the illness and consideration for other, possibly sicker patients, makes it extremely difficult to play the "consumer role" openly and without fear of criticism. Thus, self-assertion as a "client" is controlled by moral commitments to the hospital community as well as by considerations of practical and necessary self-interest.

The norms of our society permit the sick person conditionally passive withdrawal and dependence but, at the same time, emphasize the sick person's responsibility to co-operate in efforts to regain his health.[5] The prevailing image of the hospital increases the pressure to get well fast by enhancing the patient's awareness of the relative degree of the seriousness of his case. Many patients do not have to look far to find and hear about patients who seem more seriously ill. This pressure to get well also is intensified by the observation of "over-worked" and "rushed" nurses and physicians. The pattern of hospital relationships which, for the most part, prevents the development of those relationships which would reduce fears of being rejected or criticized, further discourage patients from exploiting the leniency to which illness per se may entitle them. A moral commitment to physicians and nurses is also strengthened by the gratitude and admiration of the sick for those who are "trying to help."

Patterns of interaction are also affected by the controls which the participants can exert over each other and the understanding which they can have of the function of others. For a variety of reasons, the patient sees few areas in which he has control.

A prerequisite for controlling the actions of others is the capacity to feel competent to judge their achievements. Most patients feel quite helpless in evaluating the knowledge, skill and competence of nurses and physicians. This may be one reason for their intense emphasis on "personality." "Personality" is felt to be associated with, and an indicator of, those more technical qualities which patients do not feel qualified to judge.

Control does not only depend on the capacity to judge the competence or efficiency of others. It also involves the freedom to convey and impose judgments. Even if patients feel quite certain about their judgments, they may feel reluctant to express them if such action may portend a reduction in good patient care.

The institutional context affects the way the patients balance their perceived claims and obligations. They manage to communicate the conditional nature of their claims, the undesirability of their state and, therefore, the importance of their obligations. Their persistent verbal assertions that they should co-operate, that they must not be demanding, underscore their motivation to get well. The problem of patients does not stem from a rejection of major social values but rather from the dissonance created between the desire to broaden the boundaries of what seems a legitimate sphere of control and the tendency to adhere compulsively to behavior which reflects conformity to obligations.[6] The data confirm Parsons' contention that dependence is, in our society, a primary threat to the valued achievement capacity and that the sick, to this extent, are called upon to work for their own recovery.[7]

Efforts to adhere to obligations are accompanied by the complementary hope that others will meet their obligations in turn and thus will satisfy the patient's expectations. Recognition of the limitations under which hospital functionaries work does not prevent patients from forming "ideal" expectations which call for a model of care which the on-going work processes of the hospital do not readily approximate.[8] The restraint which is exercised by the hospitalized patient is partly an expression of his fears that he may be deprived of important service if he should deviate from acceptable behavior. However, while patients have some notions of the sanctions which can be applied should they violate standards for appropriate behavior, they appear much less certain what they could do if nurses or physicians do not meet their obligations. The feeling of helplessness of patients is partly derived from an incapacity to judge adequately the competence of those who take care of them — in part, from the fact that their experiences do not provide easily defendable criteria for asserting their rights; and partly from their reluctance to use the controls which are available to them.

The interviews showed that patients always knew what they should not be like or what qualities or behavior would make them acceptable to others. Even much more difficult for them was to define what specific tasks they had a right to expect and what expectations could be transformed into active demands without deviating from general norms of behavior. A lack of familiarity with what constitutes proper care and cure procedures as well as the fact that a slight change in their condition could alter the legitimacy of demands appears to contribute to this difficulty. Rigid adherence to general rules of conduct appeared to be one way out of this dilemma.

Patients were also limited in the expression of their feelings by the fact that personalized and supportive care was not considered to lie within the sphere of the essential. They clearly felt that they had to subordinate such demands to their own or other patients' needs for physical care. The point of view of patients parallels the common distinction between the legitimacy of somatic and mental illness — a distinction which is accompanied by the notion that somatic illness legitimately entitles the ill to accept dependence as a result of manifestly impaired *physical* capacity for task performance. This dependence is narrowly defined in terms of permitting hospital functionaries to do things for the patient only as long as it is really *physically* necessary. Emotional dependence or other deviations from adult role performance are considered legitimate by most patients only in cases of extreme illness.[9]

The opportunities to obtain personalized care are limited and they are further restricted by patients who as "good patients" withdraw from those on whom they depend and with whom they wish to communicate but whom they do not wish "to bother." The control of the desire to obtain and demand more personal care tends to intensify alienation.[10] The expression of such emotional needs is checked not only by the various pressures to conform to the patient role, but also by the fact that those patient-care activities which direct themselves to the emotional needs of the patient are not institutionalized as role obligations of personnel in the general hospital. Personal concern, support or other emotionally thera-peutic efforts tend to be from the patient's point of view pleasant (often unexpected) attributes of otherwise task-oriented personnel. Such activi-ties are quickly praised and even "ideally" seen as the major attributes of the "good" nurse and of the "good" physician. But, since these do not really belong to the manifestly legitimate obligations, they are only reluctantly criticized when missing and rarely directly demanded.

Efforts to adhere to rules of conduct involve also the desire to project a specific image of self.[11] Being accepted is of more than passing importance to the hospitalized patient.[12] Self-consciousness about the norms to which one tries to conform may also suggest that the role is in certain respects alien to the performers and that they are not secure in essential social relationships. Efforts to reiterate conformity to general rules of conduct may thus, at least in part, stem from the patient's limited knowledge of the reality of the institutional setting and from fears that he may not be able to measure up to institutionalized expectations. Thus, uncertain about how far he can go before violating prescribed rules for behavior, patients may find their security in efforts to live up to the "letter of the law."[13]

The frequently expressed obligation to co-operate and the persistent attempt to seek approval is, within this frame of reference, not only a diplomatic effort to manipulate relationships to one's own advantage, but also an expression of the patient's perception of the degree of dependency associated with his status. The associated attitudes are thus not merely psychological consequences of the sick role but also reflect the patient's common sense assessments of the abrogation of independence and decision-making associated with his status in the hospital.[14] These deprivations are communicated to the patient beginning with the possessive gesture of the identification bracelet affixed during admission to the hospital, and they are continuously reinforced in daily experiences. The hospital preempts control and jurisdiction, ranging from the assumption of accountability of body functions to the withholding of information about medical procedures.[15]

The interviews reflect a degree of uncertainty whether physicians and nurses operate as effective teams in close communication or whether the patient ought to function as interpreter and intermediary between these two all important functionaries. Sometimes patients wonder whether they are sources of conflict and competition between medicine and nursing. The physician is seen as supreme authority and patients repeatedly stress that "if something is really seriously wrong," they would turn to the physician. The physician, however, is for the most part not present to observe, respond or intervene. The nurse is continually present, or at least within reach of the call system. She is the physician's representative and interpreter, but she also is the one who has to bear the brunt of work resulting from the physician's orders. She represents hospital rules, and yet she is not infrequently seen by the patient as a potential spokesman for his needs and interests. These perceptions reflect remarkably well the organization of the hospital and the ambiguous position of the nurse at the crossroads of the care and cure structures.[16]

This study suggests that the patient role, like other comparable behavior syndromes organized around a status, are not adequately described by isolating attitudinal and normative responses to the role theme itself, i.e., illness. The full repertory of role behavior must be placed into the context or organizational processes if it is to encompass realistic orientations and behavior display.

The patient role described in this paper is specific to the hospital. The data support and amplify the implication of Merton's use of the role-set as an analytic concept.[17] The patient gropes for appropriate criteria and distinctions in defining his role with reference to a variety of significant relationships. The concept points to the importance of the difference in the power of the members of the role-set *vis-à-vis* the status occupant who has to manipulate between correspondents and to the significance of the support which the status occupant receives from others in like circumstances. However, the relatively isolated patient in the modern single or double hospital room is frequently left to his own devices in coping with differences in real or perceived expectations. This adds to the conditions favoring manifestations of withdrawal or dependence on the approval of others as realistic responses to institutionalized impotence.

The data also suggests a further elaboration of certain aspects of the theoretical model of role behavior. The concept of the role-set refines the differential system of expectations attached to a status from the point of view of the range of counter roles. The data reported in this paper suggest that an additional dimension of role expectation would be a useful addition to theory. Expectations which define a role are normally attributed to the social system surrounding a status.[18] It is suggested that a distinguishable difference exists between the pattern of expectations arising from the structural aspects of the status and those expectations which are attached to the function ascribed to the role. Thus, the role concomitants of being ill can be defined as the functional role segment of the patient role while the consequences of hospitalization, be they perceived or real, could be termed positional role segments.

Concern with the functional segment of the patient role has been evidenced in most previous treatments of the sick role in the literature.[19] The positional role segment in this study is specific to the hospital. Yet in other settings for patient behavior — be it the home, the clinic or the physician's office — these structural components of the patient role would also bear fruitful sociological investigation. This conceptual scheme aids in structuring the observations of potential strain and conflict between different aspects of the patient role.

This study suggests that a prevailing theme of successful role behavior is the ability of the status occupant to integrate into his own behavior and responses different components from the system of expectations surrounding him. In the case of the patient his efforts to be "a good patient," to meet the obligations as he perceives them and to strive to co-operate in recovery are handicapped by the inadequacy of the communications system within which he functions.[20] Were it more effective, it may permit the patient to cope with his role with greater certainty about rights and obligations, the controls at his disposal and the risks inherent in behavioral experimentation.

FOOTNOTES

1. Parsons, T., "Definitions of Health and Illness in the Light of American Values and Social Structure," in E. G. Jaco (ed.), *Patients, Physicians and Illness*, New York: Free Press, 1958, pp. 165-187.

2. Thirty-two per cent of the patients in this sample occupied a private room; 61 per cent occupied a two-bed room and 7 per cent shared a room with two other patients.

3. Parsons, T., *The Social System,* New York: Free Press, 1951, pp. 433-477.

4. This phenomenon suggests a parallel to the concept of "relative deprivation" described by R. K. Merton and P. Lazarsfeld (eds.), *Continuities in Social Research,* New York: Free Press, 1950. Just as deprivation is experienced in relation to relative norms, legitimacy of claims rests on a relative basis. If this basis is not ascertainable, uncertainty functions as restraining force.

5. Parsons, T., and R. Fox, "Illness, Therapy and the Modern Urban American Family," in E. G. Jaco (ed.), *Patients, Physicians and Illness,* New York: Free Press, 1st ed., 1958, p. 236.

6. At times the patient and his significant others among hospital functionaries may be less in disagreement over proper role relationships than significant others involved in their social network. Thus, in some cases patients were found to define their obligations in terms of all the previously discussed considerations. Their relatives, however, emphasized the rights of the paying consumer and expressed their opinion that the patient was "not asking for enough." For a discussion of the role of the third party see W. J. Goode, "A Theory of Role Strain," *American Sociological Review,* 25:483-496, August, 1960.

7. Parsons, "Definitions of Health and Illness . . .," *op. cit.* p. 185.

8. Reactions to experiences in the hospital assume, therefore, meaning not only in relation to "realistic" anticipations but also in relation to more subtly held "ideal" expectations. The relative discrepancy between "realistic" and "ideal" experiences is a significant variable in the patients' responses to actual experiences.

9. Patients were not interviewed during the critical phases of their illness when, indeed, their claims may have been different. However, only a few patients in the sample considered themselves recovered. The majority of patients in the cardio-vascular category were recuperating from severe illness and were under orders for bedrest. The majority of the patients in the gastro-intestinal category were under treatment for ulcers or hospitalized for other chronic or acute gastro-intestinal conditions. In all of these cases the conditional nature of rights was bound to create some difficulties — either because of the absence of visible symptoms of illness or because the illness was not considered very serious. Case studies of the more seriously ill patients indicate that anxiety may cause them to "break through" the limits set by their role but that such a breakthrough often demands added efforts since claims, demands or irritations have to be justified. To reestablish an acceptable view of themselves seems to often constitute a major effort for these patients.

10. Parsons, "Definitions of Health and Illness . . .," *op. cit.,* p. 186. The author points out that the supportive treatment of the sick person "undercuts the alienative component of the motivational structure of his illness."

11. Goffman, E., "The Nature of Deference and Demeanor," *Amer. Anthropologist,* 58:473-502, June, 1956; E. Goffman, *Encounters: Two Studies in the Sociology of Interaction,* Indianapolis, Ind.: Bobbs-Merrill, 1961, pp. 99-105.

12. Efforts to give verbal evidence of conformity may aim at protection from criticism. Deviations tend to be viewed as forgiveable as long as a person gives evidence of "good will." Goode emphasized that failure in role behavior tends to arouse less criticism than failure in emotional commitment to general norms. This principle may be particularly applicable to situations where it is also an obligation of alters to tolerate failures in role behavior. See W. J. Goode, "Norm Commitment and Conformity to Role Status Obligations," *Amer. J. Soc.,* 66: 246-258, November, 1960.
13. See Merton's discussion of ritualism. Anxiety over the ability to live up to institutional expectations may contribute to compulsive adherence to institutional norms. R. K. Merton, *Social Theory and Social Structure,* New York: Free Press, Rev. Ed., 1957, pp. 184-187.
14. Parsons and Fox stressed the need for a "well-timed, well-chosen, well-balanced exercise of supportive and the disciplinary components of the therapeutic process." Institutional factors as well as widely held social values may tend to shift the emphasis too much to the disciplinary components particularly in the setting of the general hospital which incorporate structurally as well as in terms of explicitly or implicitly held attitudes the distinction between the emotionally sick and the physically sick (Parsons and Fox, *op.cit.,* p. 244).
15. Mauksch, H. O., "Patients View Their Roles," *Hospital Progress,* 43:136-138, October, 1962.
16. Mauksch, H. O., "The Organizational Context of Nursing Practice," in F. Davis (ed.), *The Nursing Profession,* New York: Wiley, 1966, pp. 109-137.
17. Merton, R. K., "The Role Set," *British J. Sociology,* 8:106-120, June, 1957.
18. *Ibid.,* p. 113f.
19. Parons, *The Social System, loc. cit.* Other writers, notably R. Coser, *Life in the Ward,* Lansing, Mich.: Michigan State Univ. Press, 1962, include positional considerations to a greater extent.
20. Skipper, Jr., J.K. D.L. Tagliacozzo and H. O. Mauksch, "Some Possible Consequences of Limited Communication Between Patients and Hospital Functionaries," *J. Health and Human Behavior,* 5:34-39, Spring, 1964; J. K. Skipper, Jr., "Communication and the Hospitalized Patient", in J. K. Skipper and R. C. Leonard (eds.), *Social Interaction and Patient Care,* Philadelphia: Lippincott, 1965, pp. 61-82.

Good Patients and Problem Patients: Conformity and Deviance in a General Hospital*

Judith Lorber

When a patient enters a hospital, he or she is an outsider in the health professional's place of work. Like any other workers, doctors and nurses try to arrange for their work to be conveniently and easily performed (Freidson, 1970:302-331). Hospital rules and regulations are for their benefit, not for the convenience of patients. For the sake of the smooth and efficient running of the institution, patients are categorized so they can be worked on with routines established as proper for their category. Freidson (1967) points out that rationalization, standardization, and depersonalization are felt to be "worth the price" when the results achieved clearly benefit the patient.

In order to ensure compliance even when the patient does not clearly perceive the benefits of a particular rule or regimen, doctors and nurses rely on procedures that reduce a sense of autonomy and encourage acceptance of routine treatment. A favored technique of diminishing the social status of the patient is treatment as a non-person. Goffman (1961: 341-342) describes this technique as:

> . . . the wonderful brand of "non-person treatment" found in the medical world, whereby the patient is greeted with what passes as civility, and said farewell to in the same fashion, with everything in between going on as if the patient weren't there as a social person at all, but only as a possession someone has left behind.

Cartwright (1964:95), in her study of British hospital patients, found that hospital doctors did not even bother with ordinary civilities, such as introducing themselves to patients.

The ideal situation, Goffman (1961:340-342) points out, would be to have the patient's social self go home while the damaged physical container is left for repair. But patients do come to the hospital equipped with functioning eyes, ears, and mouths, and they are in an excellent position to notice and complain about real or imagined errors, failures, inattention, and other forms of sloppiness in work that can be kept out of sight, or "backstage," when the client sees only the front office. Since many sick

From *Journal of Health and Social Behaviour*, Vol. 16, No. 2, June 1975. By permission of the author and publisher.
*This study was supported by U.S. Public Health Service Grant HS00013.

98

people in hospitals have alert periods and ample time to spy out inequities, inefficiency, and malfeasance, their possible criticisms must be neutralized. The chief method for minimizing the potentiality of patient to make trouble for doctors and nurses by criticizing their work is to withhold information, so the patient cannot argue from adequate knowledge.

The medical staff certainly does have superior knowledge and expertise for the task of treatment, and the patient can never be a true equal in this area (Freidson, 1967:497). Nevertheless, it has been argued that over and above what derives from professional expertise, doctors and nurses deliberately limit the communication of information to patients to prevent their work routines from constantly being interrupted with questions and to mask their shortcomings and failures from the scrutiny of clients who are living where they work (Brown, 1966:203; Roth, 1963a:30-59; Roth, 1963b; Skipper, 1965). In addition to shielding doctors and nurses from the criticisms of patients, limited communication protects the professional stance of detachment and concern (Davis, 1960; Quint, 1965). While the loss of personal identity seems to be the subject of vague complaints among hospital patients, explicit complaints about the difficulty of obtaining adequate information or satisfactory explanations are well-documented (Cartwright, 1964:75; Duff and Hollingshead, 1968:285-286; Lorber, 1971: Chapter VIII; Shiloh, 1965).

For the medical staff, the more like a helpless object the patient is, the easier they find it to do their job. But if the patient cannot be rendered insensate, or his or her views are ignored completely, the routinization of work is helped when the patient is objective, instrumental, emotionally neutral, completely trusting, and obedient. To Parsons' (1951:428-479), sick-role prescriptions of cooperation and motivation to get well, the hospital-patient role adds the obligations to submit to hospital routines without protest (King, 1962:355-358; Tagliacozzo and Mauksch, 1972). The result is a patient role that has the same dimensions as Parsons' (1951:428-479) professional role: it is universalistic, affectively neutral, functionally specific, and collectivity-oriented. The voluntary cooperativeness, one-to-one intimacy, and conditional permissiveness that constitutes the commonly used version of Parsons' patient role are applicable only to outpatient care by a private physician. Inpatient care imposes on patients a role characterized by submission to professional authority, enforced cooperation, and depersonalized status.

Hospitalized patients frequently resent the passivity and submission expected by doctors and nurses, yet they tend to conform. There is evidence that patients believe this is the proper way to act in a hospital; moreover, they are afraid that if they do not keep quiet and do as they are told, they may not get adequate care (Coser, 1962:80-95; Tagliacozzo and Mauksch, 1972; Skipper, 1964). Short-term patients have little recourse but conformity to what the hospital staff expects, for they are virtual loners

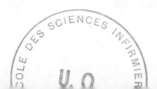

in the hospital social system. Patients usually come into the hospital singly, without a supportive group of peers. As newcomers they are on their own in learning the informal rules of the organization (Rosengren and Lefton, 1969:147-148, 156-157). If they try to buck the rules, they find no one is exclusively on their side. Other patients feel that if any one patient makes excessive demands, less attention will be paid to their own needs. Restriction of family visits effectively limits outside support of patients' demands within the hospital. Where relatives are permitted unlimited visiting, as in terminal cases, they are likely to be co-opted by the doctors and nurses to keep the patient manageable (Glaser and Strauss, 1965:92).

Although most patients accept the general norms of the hospital-patient role, Coser (1956) and Shiloh (1965) found that patients differed in their degree of acceptance. The patients Coser described as "primary" in orientation toward medical care in the hospital and Shiloh called "hierarchal" completely accept passivity, trust, and docility as proper behavior for patients. The patients Coser described as "instrumentally" oriented and Shiloh called "equalitarian" tend to reject these norms and to feel a hospitalized patient should be autonomous, critical, and well-informed. Coser did not make a systematic analysis of the behavior of these two types of patients but, on the one hand, she felt that patients who were "instrumental" tended to cause disturbances in hospital routines because they refused to give up their "substantial rationality" and were critical of the care they received. On the other hand, while "primary" patients readily adapted to ward routines, their attitudes produced the dysfunctional consequence of making them very reluctant to leave the hospital (Coser, 1956: 11-17).

Coser (1956, 1962:99-128) found that older patients tended to feel a good patient was one who was submissive to hospital rules and regulations, and Cartwright (1964:80-81) presents data that suggest that younger patients and professional and non-manual workers are somewhat aggressive in seeking information while in the hospital. Skipper (1964) found that age was a better predictor of patients' attitudes than sex or education, with those over 45 seeing themselves as having more obligations towards doctors and nurses than those under 45.

This study of hospitalized patients was undertaken to determine the variations in patients' expectations of how they should act in the hospital, to see how they actually did act during a short-term hospitalization, and to get information on the doctors' and nurses' evaluations of their behavior. It was predicted that patients who felt a good patient was one who was cooperative, trusting, uncomplaining, and undemanding would conform to these norms during their own hospital stay, while patients who did not agree with these norms would be uncooperative, argumentative, complaining, and demanding — that is, deviant from the point of view of the staff.

Research Design

The study was done at a 600-bed hospital that is part of a medical center in a bedroom borough of New York City. Patients scheduled for elective surgery were chosen as subjects because, on entering the hospital, they could be interviewed about their attitudes toward how a hospital patient should behave, and their behavior could be studied after the operation. A quota sample was selected to represent a range of seriousness of surgical procedures of ordinary enough occurence that the patients would not be singled out for special attention.

The operations were: *routine* — 33 herniorrhaphies; *moderately serious* — 26 cholecystectomies and 5 removals of polyps, masses, or benign tumors; *very serious* — 35 gastric, colon, and abdominoperineal resections, 2 caval shunts, and 2 laparotomies with biopsy. Of those who had very serious surgery, 14 did not have cancer, and 25 did. The groupings into routine, moderately serious, and very serious surgery were corroborated by medical personnel who were asked to rank seven typical procedures on extensiveness, and on amount of medical attention, nursing care, and reassurance they felt were needed by the patient.

The 103 patients on whom data were collected were fairly equally divided by sex. By age, 16 percent were under 40, 17 percent were 41-50, 26 percent were 51-60, and 42 percent were over 60. (Percentages are rounded.) Their educational attainment was low: 39 percent had not graduated from high school, 36 percent were high school graduates and 25 percent had some college or were college graduates. They were predominantly Jewish: 60 percent; 24 percent were Catholic, 11 percent were Anglo-Saxon Protestant, 7 percent were other. Ethnic-religious groups were based on the birth-place or self or father, where foreign-born, of self and father where American-born, and own religion. Anglo-Saxon Protestants included those whose own and/or father's birthplace was the United States, England, Scotland, Scandinavia, or Canada.

In order to find out their attitudes about how a hospital patient should act, on the day of admission or immediately after they were informed they would be having surgery, patients were asked to agree, agree strongly, disagree, or disagree strongly with six statements. In the following statements, agreement indicated conforming attitudes.

Doctors expect patients to obey them completely.

The sicker a patient is, the more attention he or she can expect from the doctors and the nurses.

The best thing to do in the hospital is to keep quiet and do what you're told.

In the following statements, disagreement indicated conforming attitudes:

I cooperate best as a patient when I know the reason for what I have to do.

When I'm sick I expect to be pampered and catered to.

It would be nice to talk to my nurse about any family or personal problems I had.

In the final analysis, all the "agree" responses and all the "disagree" responses were grouped in order to increase the size of the cell N's. The patients were categorized as having very conforming, moderately conforming, and deviant attitudes according to the number of their conforming responses. The number of conforming responses per group were: *very conforming* — 6 (4 patients), 5 (29 patients); *moderately conforming* — 4 (42 patients); *deviant* — 3 (18 patients), 2 (8 patients), 1 (2 patients). The cutting points were set at what seemed natural breaks to create groups of roughly equal size.

The responses to a self-administered questionnaire distributed to the doctors and nurses who had cared for the patient supplied data on *their* evaluations of the patients. The questionnaire was filled out at the end of the patient's stay in the hospital, or shortly after the patient had been discharged.

Conforming and Deviant Attitudes

Between men and women, there was little difference in attitudes toward the hospital-patient role. By ethnic-religious group, American-born Catholics tended to have deviant attitudes, while Anglo-Saxon Protestants and Irish Catholics tended to have very conforming attitudes. However, the ethnic-religious groupings were so skewed that these findings are merely suggestive. Age and education did have an effect on attitudes toward the hospital-patient role. The younger and better educated the patient, the less likely he or she was to express very conforming attitudes. The highest percentage of patients with very conforming attitudes was found among the elderly high school graduates. Very few of the poorly educated patients of any age expressed deviant attitudes. Among the college-educated, those under 60 tended to express deviant attitudes, and those over 60 to be moderately conforming in their attitudes.

It might be expected that the more serious the illness, the less likely the patient would be to express deviant attitudes, since the sicker patients would feel more dependent on doctors and nurses than those about to undergo routine procedures, or be too weak to be assertive. While the highest percentage of patients with very conforming attitudes was among those who had cancer, the next highest was among those who had routine hernia repairs, and the difference in percentages was very small. On the other hand, almost half the very serious surgery patients who did not have cancer had deviant attitudes, compared to about one-quarter of the patients having all the types of procedures. The herniorrhaphy patients, having been warned that the whole procedure was quite routinized, may have felt they had little to gain by insisting on their autonomy, while the cancer patients may have been scared by the ambiguities of the information they were given. (One woman, whose tumor really turned out to be benign, did not believe her surgeon was telling her the truth.) The very serious surgery patients who did not have cancer were among the best-informed patients, since they came to surgery usually after a long history of medically-treated illness. However, their extensive experience with medical settings had not overly socialized them into accepting the professional's model of the "good patient."

In this study, then, the best predictors of deviant or conforming attitudes toward the hospital-patient role were age and education. As the population gets better educated, and the social distance between lay people and professionals narrows, it is likely that patients will probably be asking more questions, demanding more explicit information about their cases, and insisting on more personalized attention.

Conforming and Deviant Behavior

A direct manifestation of acceptance or rejection of the norm of compliance is the extent to which a patient will argue about prescribed routines. In the interview given just before discharge, patients were asked if they had refused to follow a doctor's or nurse's order or questioned or complained about one. Of the 98 patients who answered the question about doctors, 24 percent said they had disagreed with doctors (mostly house staff and known as such to the patients). Of the 99 patients who answered the question about nurses, 18 percent said they had disagreed with nurses. The arguments were mostly over medication, tests, procedures, mechanical devices, and coughing (cf. Davis and Von der Lippe, 1968).

Patients with deviant attitudes, who did not subscribe to the norm of unquestioning obedience, had been expected to disagree more than patients with conforming attitudes. While only slightly more than one-third of the patients with deviant attitudes disagreed with either doctors or nurses, they did have the highest percentages of those disagreeing, as predicted. As Table 1 shows, patients with very conforming attitudes tended to disagree least, and patients with moderately conforming attitudes were midway between. In open confrontation, the association of attitudes with behavior was clearly in the predicted direction.

An ambiguous source of conflict between patients and medical staff is complaints of pain and discomfort. A certain amount of complaining is expected by doctors and nurses — the acceptable amount being determined by the extensiveness of the surgical procedure, the age and sex of the patient, and the ethnic group of doctor or nurse (Zborowski, 1969). Since the acceptable level varies so, complaints of physical discomfort can be used by hospital patients as subtle weapons of conflict and as a means of getting attention. Therefore, it was predicted that patients who accepted "good-patient" norms would be likely to complain less than patients whose attitudes were deviant.

In all the types of surgery studied, patients with deviant attitudes had the highest percentage of those who complained a great deal about minor discomforts, such as nausea, gas pains, insomnia, headache, and lassitude. In routine and moderately serious surgery, patients with very conforming attitudes had the lowest percentage of complainers, but in very serious surgery, patients with moderately conforming attitudes had the lowest percentage of complainers. In short, patients with very conforming attitudes tended to complain comparatively less and patients with deviant attitudes tended to complain comparatively more no matter how serious their illness, while patients with moderately conforming attitudes seemed to complain according to how much attention was paid them. In routine surgery, where they got little attention, they had almost as high a percentage of complainers as patients with deviant attitudes. In very serious surgery, where they got a great deal of attention, they had the lowest percentage of complainers.

According to these data, most hospital patients comply unquestioningly with doctors' and nurses' orders and limit their complaints, but patients with deviant views of their role tend to argue with the medical staff and to register frequent minor complaints. The question to be explored now is what the medical staff's reaction was to conforming and deviant patients.

TABLE 1.   DISAGREEMENTS WITH STAFF, BY PATIENTS' ATTITUDES

	Patients' Attitudes		
Disagreements with Doctors[a]:	% Very Conforming (N=32)	% Moderately Conforming (N=39)	% Deviant (N=27)
Never Disagreed	88	74	63
Disagreed	13	26	37
Disagreements with Nurses[b]:	% Very Conforming (N=32)	% Moderately Conforming (N=39)	% Deviant (N=28)
Never Disagreed	94	85	64
Disagreed	6	15	36

[a] Five patients did not answer this question.
[b] Four patients did not answer this question.

Good, Average, and Problem Patients

From nurses' description of patients, Duff and Hollingshead (1968:221-222, their emphasis) concluded that patients were divided into two categories — "problem" and "no problem." As they put it, "The definition of a *problem* is related to the degree to which the patient needed physical care or was unable to comply with orders." In other words, ". . . *problem* patients obstructed work and *no problem* patients facilitated work." In this study, the doctors' and nurses' choice of "good patient," "average patient," or "problem patient" on the self-administered questionnaire they were asked to fill out at the end of the patients' stay, plus their invited remarks on the questionnaire and in private conversation with the researcher, all bore out the relationship between the label of good or problem patient and the extent to which the patient made trouble for them. Patients who were considered cooperative, uncomplaining, and stoical by the doctors and nurses were generally labeled good patients, no matter what their procedure or postoperative complications.

For instance, the private-duty nurse who spent 36 nights caring for a young woman with extensive postoperative complications following a gallbladder removal wrote: ". . . A very good patient to my way of thinking because no matter how much pain, she was always pleasant and not disagreeable. She *tried at all times* [sic] to be cooperative even though the tension in her was great at all times." After 29 consecutive days of nursing a 55-year-old man who had a shunt operation for cirrhosis of the liver followed by almost fatal complications, the private-duty nurse said, "I really enjoyed taking care of him. He was never grouchy, always cooperative — even though he was sick." In talking of a 63-year-old woman who was vice-president of her local chapter of Cancer Care, and who had an extensive operation for cancer, her surgeon said to the researcher, "You sent me a questionnaire on the most cooperative patient I've seen in 35 years. . . . She had massive surgery — she had complications — but she never complains. She knows she had a malignancy, but she doesn't have to be reassured — she says, 'The axe had to fall sometime.' "

In contrast, patients whom the doctors and nurses felt were uncooperative, constantly complaining, overemotional, and dependent were frequently considered problem patients, whether they had routine or very serious surgery. For example, the resident and intern labeled a problem patient a 62-year-old man who had a hernia repair with no complications, but who had been extremely apprehensive about the operation. In the patient's medical record, the resident noted that he was "overreacting to his condition," and had "multiple complaints related to his personality." The intern simply called him *"a kvetch."* A 74-year-old man who had a gallbladder removal with many postoperative complications, some psychosomatic, was labeled a problem patient by the surgeon, resident, intern, and day staff nurse. In the questionnaire, the resident said the patient's uncooperativeness made it difficult to perform routine procedures on him. The surgeon wrote that the patient was "lachrymose, combative, and generally impossible." To the researcher, the surgeon added that the patient had called him names, lied, and generally carried on.

Another patient considered a problem patient by her surgeon, the day staff nurse, and a private-duty nurse (but a good patient by the intern) was a pretty, 30-year-old divorcee. She told everyone about her family problems and described herself as a "devout coward." She had an uncomplicated gallbladder removal, but cried a lot and was given tranquilizers. The day head nurse said of her, "This patient seemed to have been pampered very much. She barely cooperated and seemed to have been extremely dependent on her mother. She was much more of a baby than most people having the same surgery."

The doctors and nurses on a case frequently did not agree on the evaluation of the patient. The same patient could be labeled good, problem, and average, and no patient was labeled a problem by every doctor or nurse who returned a questionnaire on him or her. The doctor or nurse who bore the brunt of the difficulty was usually the one who considered the patient a problem patient, while the others labeled him or her good or average. This supports the original contention that problem patients were those who created trouble for the medical staff.

A case in point was a young, well-educated man with a wife and child who was discovered to have a fast-growing, inoperable, and extremely painful form of cancer. He was very agitated before and after surgery, and he was demanding after surgery. But only the resident, with whom he fought over the question of pain medication, labeled him a problem patient. The resident said of him, "Very argumentative about getting his own way." The patient needed little physical care, so the rest of the staff was able, in the words of the head nurse, to "humor him." The private-duty nurse on the case, a young woman, refused to fill out a questionnaire but told me, "I couldn't stand the man." She felt he was tyrannical and he thought her incompetent. With him for twelve hours a day, she would, of course, have borne the brunt of his troublesome behavior.

TABLE 2.   MEDICAL STAFF EVALUATIONS, BY PATIENTS' ATTITUDES[a]

Staff Evaluations		% Very Conforming (N=33)	% Moderately Conforming (N=42)	% Deviant (N=28)
Attending	Good	67	74	64
Physician	Problem	3	5	14
Resident	Good	36	41	46
	Problem	6	7	11
Intern	Good	46	52	36
	Problem	3	7	11
Day Staff	Good	33	38	39
Nurse	Problem	3	7	14

[a]Omits those labeled "average" and "no answer." Non-return of a questionnaire is an indication that the patient did not register one way or another; in general, the doctors and nurses were more inclined to fill out questionnaires for patients they either admired or found troublesome.

It was reported earlier that, while most patients were obedient and uncomplaining, patients with deviant attitudes toward the hospital-patient role were more argumentative and complained more than patients with conforming attitudes. Did the doctors and nurses more often label patients with deviant attitudes problem patients? Although the percentage differences were not large, they were in the expected direction: patients with deviant attitudes were most often labeled problem patients by the time they left the hospital, patients with moderately conforming attitudes less frequently, and patients with very conforming attitudes least of all. (See Table 2.)

Note, however, that very conforming patients were not labeled *good* patients to any great degree. One consequence of their uncomplaining, passive behavior might have been that they did not ask for help when they really needed it, so the nurses had to take time to do frequent checks on their physical status. For instance, a nurse wrote in the questionnaire of a 62-year-old woman who had very extensive abdominal surgery and was herself a nurse, "This patient was far too considerate of the nurses . . . she 'didn't want to bother' us and often remained quiet when in pain and had to be frequently checked for comfort." The nurse's use of quotation marks around the phrase "didn't want to bother" highlights the point that by not asking for needed attention, the patient, who should have known better, disrupted the usual routine. In this way the too stoical or too passive patient can also cause trouble.

Routine Management and Extraordinary Trouble

The analysis of the doctors' and nurses' evaluations of patients suggested that ease of management was the basic criterion for a label of good patient, and that patients who took time and attention felt to be unwarranted by their illness tended to be labeled problem patients. Robert Emerson (1971) points out that those troublemakers who can be managed routinely by social control agents are treated relatively leniently; only those who do not let themselves be managed routinely — who need extraordinary solutions to their problems — are singled out for stronger sanctions.

In the hospital studied, the medical staff expected a certain amount of complaining from surgical patients, particularly about pain. The most frequently mentioned method of handling *any* complaint was the use of sedative or narcotic drugs. Sixty-nine percent of the 499 questionnaires returned by the doctors and nurses mentioned drugs as the method used to handle complaints. The next most popular method was mentioned in only 34 percent of the returned questionnaires; it was talking to patients — reassuring, encouraging, explaining, ordering, scolding, and so on. Physical methods, such as turning, positioning, walking around, examining, making comfortable, and so on, were mentioned in 22 percent of the returned questionnaires, and methods that used mechanical devices were listed in 14 percent. (Mentions were multiple.) All the less favored methods took more time than the administration of a shot or oral dose of pain reliever or sedative every four hours.

Negative evaluations of relatively high percentages of patients who took up more time and were talked to fit in with the medical staff's own designation of which were the usual and which the less common methods of managing complaints. When the reports of amount of time spent with patients were cross-tabulated with evaluations of the patients, it was found that the patients with whom more time was spent were much more likely to be labeled problem patients than those with whom average or less than average time was spent. The doctors labeled as problem patients from 25 to 36 percent of those they said took up more than the usual amount of time for that type of surgery. Between 80 and 91 percent of the patients the doctors said took up less than the average amount of time for their type of surgery were labeled good patients. In short, the less of the doctor's time the patient took, the better he or she was viewed.

Similarly, doctors and nurses were more likely to label problem patients those they remembered having talked to, and less likely to label them good patients. Residents and day staff nurses, who had the responsibility for the daily management of the surgical wards, labeled as problem patients one-quarter of those they singled out as having been talked to. (See Table 3.)

TABLE 3.   MEDICAL STAFF EVALUATIONS OF PATIENTS, BY REPORTS OF TALKING TO PATIENTS[a]

Staff Evaluations		Questionnaire Responses	
		% Reporting Talk	% Reporting No Talk
Attending		N=20	N=71
Physician	Good	60	83
	Problem	10	7
Resident		N=29	N=44
	Good	45	66
	Problem	24	2
Intern		N=32	N=45
	Good	41	76
	Problem	13	7
Day Staff		N=25	N=46
Nurse	Good	36	63
	Problem	24	4

[a]Omits those labeled "average" and "no answer."

The assumption that problem patients would be those who gave doctors and nurses the most trouble was borne out by other data, namely, the evaluations of patients having different types of procedures. Hernia-repair patients, who were so easy to care for they were virtually anonymous to the interns, residents, and nurses, were rarely labeled problem patients. Patients who had gallbladders removed or other moderately serious surgery, were most often described as problem patients by attending surgeons, residents and interns. Though medically routine, the post-operative condition of these patients called for a lot of attention, most of which was the residents' responsibility. It is not surprising that residents labeled as good patients only 19 percent of the moderately serious surgery cases. (See Table 4)

TABLE 4.   MEDICAL STAFF EVALUATIONS OF PATIENTS, BY SURGICAL PROCEDURE[a]

Staff *Evaluations*		% Routine (N=33)	% Moderately Serious (N=31)	% Very Serious No Cancer (N=14)	% Very Serious Cancer (N=25)
			Type of Procedure		
Attending Physician	Good	76	65	71	64
	Problem	3	10	7	8
Resident	Good	46	19	43	60
	Problem	6	13	0	8
Intern	Good	39	36	64	56
	Problem	3	16	7	0
Day Staff Nurse	Good	42	29	36	40
	Problem	0	13	14	8

[a]Omits those labeled "average" and "no answer."

To summarize, there are two variables involved in whether a doctor or nurse in charge views the patient a manageable by routine methods or as needing extraordinary solutions taking more time and attention. Patients manageable by routine methods are average — they make ordinary, expected trouble. These patients have routine illnesses, no post-operative complications, are moderately cooperative, and only occasionally complain of pain or discomfort. (Some staff members labeled them good patients, especially if they couldn't remember them too well.) Patients who might be expected to cause extraordinary trouble because of the problematic nature of their illness, but who only cause ordinary trouble because of their extraordinary cooperativeness and cheerful stoicism, are frequently rewarded with the accolade "good patient" by doctors and nurses who do not ordinarily use that label, and "great patient" by the rest.

As for those labeled problem patients, they are of two types. The first has an ordinary illness but takes up more time and attention than is warranted by the medical condition because he or she is uncooperative and/or complains and argues much of the time. Doctors and nurses consider such behavior unnecessary and therefore extraordinary trouble, and the patient is soundly condemned. The second type of problem patient has an extraordinary medical status, such as severe complications, poor prognosis, or difficult diagnosis. Troublesome behavior of the sort described above, while not approved of, is somewhat forgiven as understandable given the patient's medical condition. The first kind of problem patient seems to be considered deliberately deviant — willfully causing extraordinary trouble; the second kind of problem patient seems to be considered an accidental deviant — responding with troublesome behavior to an extraordinarily difficult situation beyond his or her control (cf. Lorber, 1967).

Possible Consequences of Being Labeled A Problem Patient

What do doctors and nurses do about those patients whose deviant behavior hinders their efficient routines? In the study reported here, patients whose behavior was troublesome and who did not respond to tranquilizers or sedation were sent home or recommended to a convalescent center where the nurses were trained to do psychotherapy. In one case, a staff psychiatrist was asked to see a troublesome dying patient who had been in psychiatric treatment before his illness. In short, deviant behavior on the part of these mostly middle-class, paying, short-term surgical patients was treated moderately permissively by the medical professionals who cared for them.

Indeed, the hospital tried various ways to meet the socio-emotional needs of its patients. A "patient-relations nurse coordinator" had been appointed for the general surgical wards for a short time before this research was done. This role was modeled after the "clinical nurse specialist" who worked closely with the open-heart surgeon. (See Bandman, Wolpin, and Rehm, 1964.) On the general surgery wards, where there were many more attending surgeons and their patients to contend with, this nurse-liaison did not work out. It was said in personal communication during preliminary fieldwork that the medical personnel felt she was spying on them, while the patients did not feel their complaints were taken care of adequately.

Another short-lived experiment that took place just after the fieldwork was done was to allow all patients on the surgical wards the same all-day visiting hours as the private-room patients. This attempt to give patients additional support lasted about two months. Given the fact that with regular visiting hours, more complaints by patients were reported on the staff questionnaires by the evening staff nurses than any other shift (evening visits were the most popular), it is probable that patient-staff conflict was exacerbated, not eased, by the constant presence of relatives.

Other studies have found that the troublesome patient tends to be somewhat neglected by the medical staff. Interns have admitted giving "superior care to the better liked, with minimum but adequate care to those not liked" (Daniels, 1960:263). Those not liked were patients who tended to be complaining and uncooperative and to ask a lot of questions. Responding to hypothetical situations, 40 nurses said they would do more for the non-complaint patient in the short run, but in the long run, predicted they would do more for the complaint patient (Keller, 1971). In their study of dying patients, Glaser and Strauss (1965) found that nurses scolded, reprimanded, and then avoided those patients who asked a lot of questions, created emotional scenes, or refused to cooperate with hospital routines. Roth and Eddy (1967: 106-109), in their study of rehabilitation patients, noted that abusive and uncooperative patients were discharged from the ward, and thus denied retraining. However, young patients with a greater chance of successful rehabilitation than older ones were treated more leniently. Roth's (1963a:41) research on long-term tuberculosis patients showed that "noisy agitation" sometimes resulted in slightly earlier discharge, especially if the staff felt the patient might leave against medical advice. But he also found hospitals with locked wards for "recalcitrant" patients whose medical status was still poor (Roth, 1963a:25). The rare cooperative and cured patient who didn't want to leave the hospital left the staff in a complete quandry, and a psychiatrist was used as a last resort (Roth, 1963a:48).

Of all these responses to extraordinarily troublesome patients, the use of psychiatrists has the most potentially momentous consequences. Meyer and Mendelson (1961) studied 60 requests for psychiatric consultation with patients on medical and surgical wards, and found that a disruptive patient was first considered uncooperative or bad, but then defined as irrational and irresponsible, or "crazy," and a psychiatrist was called in. If a patient refuses to submit quietly to hospital routines and is referred to a psychiatrist because of disruptive behavior, he or she is labeled as someone with psychiatric problems. If the fact that he or she had seen a psychiatrist is entered into the medical records, the information becomes a permanent part of his or her future identity as a patient for all other professionals who have access to this set of records. His or her future behavior will be interpreted in the light of the putative psychiatric problems, and any opposition to the way he or she is treated will never be taken seriously. Even if the information is not officially recorded, ward scuttlebut will certainly spread the word around — problem patients are discussed *ad infinitum.* For the remainder of the particular hospitalization, the patient will be treated as psychotic or neurotic, and not as someone with possible legitimate complaints (cf. Phillips, 1963, and Rosenhan, 1973).

Summary

On the basis of an attitude questionnaire administered to 103 surgical patients before their operations, this study found that most general-hospital patients enter the hospital feeling they should be obedient, cooperative, objective about their illness, and expect attention only if they are very ill. As other researchers have found, the better educated and younger patients tended to have more autonomous or deviant attitudes toward being a hospital patient. This study found that patients with deviant attitudes tended to argue more with the residents, interns, and nurses, and to complain more about minor discomforts as a way of getting attention. Although patients feel that doctors and nurses always approve of obedience, cooperation, and undemandingness, a questionnaire administered to the medical staff at the end of the patients' stay in the hospital revealed that the staff's evaluations of the patients under their care depended on the amount of trouble these patients gave them. In general, cooperative, uncomplaining, and stoical patients *were* considered good patients, but the staff expected patients to make them aware of their needs; that is, to ask for attention when it was needed medically. Patients whom the doctors and nurses felt were uncooperative, overemotional, and who complained when it was not medically warranted were considered problem patients only by the staff member who had to bear the brunt of the trouble. Patients who did not respond to sedation or tranquilizers — the chief methods of handling complaints of pain and discomfort — but instead had to be reassured, encouraged, given explanations or exhortations, and who therefore took up more of the staff's time than they felt warranted by the extent of surgery, were also considered problem patients to a greater degree than those who took up an "average" amount of time and attention.

Patients who had the most routine surgery were usually labeled good patients, as were the very cooperative seriously ill patients. The patients who had surgery that is major and painful by lay standards, but routine by medical standards, were labeled problem patients to the greatest degree, particularly by the residents, who were primarily responsible for their care. (In this study, most of these patients were, in the doctors' words, "well-nourished" middle-aged women, which may have added to the impatience the residents, both male and female, showed with them.)

In sum, doctors and nurses expect to carry out their work by well-established routines, with a minimum of interruption from patients. Those patients who make no trouble at all, who do not interrupt the smoothness of medical routines, are likely to be considered *good* patients by the medical staff. In this study, good patients usually had routine surgery and were out of the hospital within a week, or had uncomplicated major surgery and accepted whatever was done to them cheerfully and cooperatively. Doctors and nurses tend to consider *average* patients those whose complaints are medically warranted, who respond to established routines for handling such complaints, and who therefore take up the expected amount of time for their type of illness. In this study, most of the average patients had uncomplicated major surgery, complained a fair amount about pain and discomfort, but were satisfied when their requests for attention were answered with pain medication every four hours for two or three days.

Problem patients are of two kinds. Those who are seriously ill, and who complain a great deal, are very emotional, anxious, and need a lot of reassurance, encouragement, and attention from the staff are problematic, but "forgiveable" because the situation is not of their own making. In this study, they were often given the time and attention they demanded, particularly if they were grateful for it. Nonetheless, the extraordinary amount of time and attention they took up made them "problem patients." (Conversely, seriously ill patients who were extraordinarily cheerful cooperative, uncomplaining, and objective about their illness were considered *great* patients and talked about after discharge as "ideal.") Patients who are *not* seriously ill in the staff's eyes, but who nevertheless act as if they are by complaining, crying, and refusing to cooperate with medical routines, are the most soundly condemned by the staff. Such problem patients, in this study, were tranquilized, sometimes discharged early, and, in one case, referred to a psychiatrist — types of response to wilfully troublesome patients other researchers have also found.

Thus, the consequences of deliberate deviance in the general hospital can be medical neglect or a stigmatizing label, while conformity to good-patient norms is usually a return home with only a surgical scar.

BIBLIOGRAPHY

Bandman, E., S. Wolpin and D. Rehm.
1964 "The patient-relations nurse coordinator." American Journal of Nursing 64 (September): 133-135.

Brown, Esther Lucile.
1966 "Nursing and patient care." Pp. 176-203 in Fred Davis (ed.) The Nursing Profession. New York: Wiley.

Cartwright, Ann.
1964 Human Relations and Hospital Care. London: Routledge and Kegan Paul.

Coser, R.L.
1956 "A home away from home." Social Problems 4 (July): 3-17.
1962 Life in the Ward. East Lansing: Michigan State University Press.

Daniels, M.J.
1960 "Affect and its control in the medical intern." American Journal of Sociology 61 (November): 259-267.

Davis, F.
1960 "Uncertainty in medical prognosis, clinical and functional." American Journal of Sociology 66 (July): 41-47.

Davis, M.S. and R.P. von der Lippe.
1968 "Discharge from hospital against medical advice: A study of reciprocity in the doctor-patient relationship." Social Science and Medicine 1: 336-342.

Duff, Raymond S. and August B. Hollingshead.
1968 Sickness and Society. New York: Harper and Row.

Emerson, Robert M.
1971 "Trouble and unmanageability: Working notes on social control and practical action." Unpublished manuscript.

Freidson, Eliot.
  1966   "Disability as social deviance." Pp. 71-99 in Marvin B. Sussman (ed.), Sociology and Rehabilitation. Washington D.C.: American Sociological Association.
  1967   "Review essay: Health factories, the new industrial sociology." Social Problems 14 (Spring): 493-500.
  1970   Profession of Medicine. New York: Dodd, Mead.

Glaser, Barney G. and Anselm L. Strauss.
  1965   Awareness of Dying. Chicago: Aldine.

Goffman, Erving.
  1961   Asylums. Garden City, New York: Doubleday Anchor.

Keller, N.S.
  1971   "Compliance, previous access and provision of services by registered nurses." Journal of Health and Social Behavior 12 (December): 321-330.

King, Stanley H.
  1962   Perceptions of Illness and Medical Practice. New York: Russell Sage Foundation.

Lorber, J.
  1967   "Deviance as performance: The case of illness." Social Problems 14 (Winter): 302-310.
  1971   Going Under the Knife: A Study of the Sick Role in the Hospital. Unpublished Ph.D. Thesis. New York: New York University.

Meyer, E. and M. Mendelson.
  1961   "Psychiatric consultations with patients on medical and surgical wards: Patterns and processes." Psychiatry 24 (August): 197-220.

Parsons, Talcott.
  1951   The Social System. Glencoe: Free Press.

Phillips, D.L.
  1963   "Rejection: A possible consequence of seeking help for mental disorders." American Sociological Review 28 (December): 963-972.

Quint, J.C.
  1965   "Institutionalized practices of information control." Psychiatry 28 (May): 119-132.

Rosengren, William R. and Mark Lefton.
  1969   Hospitals and Patients. New York: Atherton.

Rosenhan, D.L.
  1973   "On being sane in insane places." Science 179 (January 19): 250-258.

Roth, Julius A.
1963a Timetables: Structuring the Passage of Time in Hospital Treatment and Other Careers. Indianapolis: Bobbs-Merrill.
1963b "Information and the control of treatment in tuberculosis hospitals." Pp. 293-318 in Eliot Freidson (ed.), The Hospital in Modern Society. New York: Free Press.

Roth, Julius A. and Elizabeth M. Eddy.
1967 Rehabilitation for the Unwanted. New York: Atherton.

Shiloh, A.
1965 "Equalitarian and hierarchal patients: An investigation among Hadassah Hospital patients." Medical Care 3 (April-June): 87-95.

Skipper, James K., Jr.
1964 The Social Obligations of Hospitalized Patients: A System Analysis. Unpublished Ph.D. Thesis. Evanston: Northwestern University.
1965 "Communication and the hospitalized patient." Pp. 61-82 in James K. Skipper, Jr., and Robert C. Leonard (eds.), Social Interaction and Patient Care. Philadelphia: J.B. Lippincott.

Tagliacozzo, Daisy L. and Hans O. Mauksch.
1972 "The patient's view of the patient's role." Pp. 172-185 in E. Gartly Jaco (ed.), Patients, Physicians and Illness. Second Edition. New York: Free Press.

Zborowski, Mark.
1969 People in Pain. San Francisco: Jossey-Bass.

Gaining Awareness of Cultural Difference: A Case Example

Raphella Sohier

It is my opinion that the type of understanding which we call science can begin anywhere, at any level of sophistication. To observe acutely, to think carefully and creatively — these activities, not the accumulation of laboratory instruments, are the beginnings of science.[9]

During the last few years a core of nurse-anthropologists in the United States have given leadership to the development of the subfield Leininger[6] calls "transcultural nursing." This subfield had been generally ignored or perceived to be of little importance as a systematic field of study in nursing and health care. Growing interest in this essential area of study in contemporary nursing care is encouraging. A pioneer in the field, Leininger[3] states, "It needs active attention in research and educational endeavors." In one of her several works on the subject[5], she asks the critical question: "Is it possible for an outsider who is not a member of that culture to become a helping person in a kin-based community?" This paper will address this question by using a case example to demonstrate the phenomenon of cultural awareness and the transcultural nursing process and its implications.

Awareness of certain phenomenon can frequently develop quite independently in different parts of the world. It is of interest that at the time Leininger and other colleagues were laying the groundwork for the new subfield of transcultural nursing in the U.S.A., I was striving to find solutions to problems of a transcultural nature in Belgium in 1969 and 1970. My discovery of the importance of the nurse's having an understanding of cultural factors in patient care seemed extremely important and unique. Since that time Leininger has published a book on the general subject of culture and nursing, is preparing another book, and has written many articles and given talks on the subject of transcultural nursing care since 1963. She has stressed the need to develop a body of transcultural nursing theory and concomitant skills to facilitate the delivery of optimal care to people of different cultures. Her writings provide a clear picture of nursing education's deficits in regard to cultural theory and the barriers to the acquisition of transcultural skills and knowledge. Most importantly, she contends that transcultural nursing is a legitimate field of specialized study and should be an essential part of all nursing and health care practices.

Unquestionably, many nurses working with patients whose cultural backgrounds differ from theirs, feel varying degrees of inadequacy in

From *Transcultural Health Care Issues & Conditions*, edited by Madeleine Leininger, F.A. Davis Company, 1976. By permission of the author and publisher.

sensitively handling patients' cultural needs and problems. Patients outside of the dominant culture have often expressed their feelings that nurses do not comprehend their situation, needs, and concerns. Health care projects at home and abroad have often failed or had minimal success which makes one realize that goodwill is not an adequate criterion for success in transcultural health projects. "Doc adapts modern medicine to the customs of the Cakchiquel. He feels that too often well-meaning missionary and other organized groups fail, precisely because they have tried to do it the other way round."[1] Few nurses have been prepared in the field of anthropology, but a growing number are awakening to the need for such knowledge. The fields of anthopology and nursing are quite complimentary, and this has been well documented in the writings of Osborne[7] and Leininger.[5]

A Case Study

THE BEGINNING OF AWARENESS

I went in 1958 to live and work in Belgium. Having completed a program of study in nursing, I was ready to help others as a professional nurse. At this time I became aware of the need for transcultural nursing knowledge and skills. In the case study which follows I will explicate the development of transcultural awareness and the important place of cultural values in the provision of comprehensive nursing care, clarifying what occurred in a reciprocal nurse-patient transcultural experience over a span of time. Personal values, the subculture of nursing, patient values and attitudes, and psycho-physical therapeutic care process will be highlighted. Indeed, mutual learning occurred, which provided one of the richest nursing experiences in my life and altered the course of my professional goals to focus more on transcultural nursing.

THE SCOTTISH NURSE AND NURSING EDUCATION

Nursing education in Scotland in the 1950s was moving toward a new focus, and although it has not yet attained the degree of academic excellence of American nursing at university level, still the quality of nursing education and expectations were noteworthy. The average graduate of the Scottish nursing program emerged as a competent and confident nurse who was ready to learn new ideas. Accordingly, I envisioned myself as a competent and intelligent nurse with a desire to learn more about patient care.

When I went to live in Belgium, I brought my Scottish heritage and its subculture of nursing. My Scottish culture emphasized the values of equality, social justice, honesty, and industry. The subculture of nursing in

Scotland emphasized the values of personalized care, support and respect of human dignity with ethical practices, and the right of every human being to receive quality health care. Nurses were viewed with respect and even with awe. Babies were delivered by midwives with a high level of competence and their independent performance was not only accepted but expected. District nurses had cars, as did health visitors (community health nurses), which gave them a high degree of independence. In general, the nurse was viewed as having a spotless character or, if otherwise, the ideal values of Florence Nightingale in her public and professional endeavors.

I was born in Edinburgh, Scotland, and was socialized in a Scottish Presbyterian home. Our family culture was a highly disciplined one, but love was shared not only within the family and among friends but with all people as brothers. Racial prejudice was not evident. Family members were taught that other families lived differently and this idea was accepted and recognized.

As the only daughter, I was encouraged from an early age to choose an excellent profession, namely, nursing. I was not actively discouraged from pursuing other directions, and medical school was another possibility. I envisioned no great barriers to the delivery of optimal nursing care beyond that of language. Fortunately, my nursing instruction had stressed the importance of the patient as a total person with individual needs, and so I was aware that generalized care alone was not sufficient. Personalized care with careful observation and the ability to recognize conflict and different needs was part of my way of operating as a professional nurse.

THE PROBLEM

With these values and self-perception, I began working for the first time in my life in a large Jewish community. A few days were essential to recognize my own distress signals and my need to adjust to a new cultural group, the Jewish people. Indeed, these people appeared strange and different to me. I did not comprehend their values and behavior for some time, even when they spoke excellent English. I knew, however, that I was not meeting the needs of the Jewish family. While my nursing school in Scotland had taught me to provide physiological and psychological care to patients, this was not enough. I could not read their family signals, nor distinguish clearly between physiological and psychological needs of the people in relation to their cultural orientation and values. These Jewish people seemed overly solicitous of themselves, fearful, demanding, and unusually insecure. I could not understand why they did not respond to nursing practices which ordinarily brought favorable results in Scotland. Curiosity and professional idealism combined and I began to see the challenge as well as the reasons why this family was not being understood. Thus, the problem of understanding and responding to this new Jewish culture became evident as a real challenge.

A NEW CULTURE TO THE NURSE

The Jewish community in Antwerp is very large and most of its members are traditional; some people are deeply religious and others less so. Most of the Jewish people are of Eastern European origin and use the customs of the traditional Shtetl communities which had their origin in Russia, Poland, and Hungary.[14] Almost all of these people speak several languages, an average being five.

After a few nursing encounters, I tried to evaluate the needs of the Jewish patients but found my lack of knowledge a barrier to understanding the people. In general, the most direct manner of learning about a culture is to become what anthropologists call a participant observer. So when I started as a private duty nurse to assist a Jewish gentleman in his home, I had a unique opportunity to become a participant observer and learn firsthand the patient's culture, values, and lifeways in his familial environment.

Toshek, the patient I came to know, was a 54-year-old diamond merchant who had a history of a recent, severe myocardial infarction and an aortic aneurysm. He suffered recurrent episodes of angina which were not always relieved by medication, and his prognosis was poor. I recognized the opportunity to take care of this man as a privilege and challenge and went to his home on the first day with apprehension. While attending to Toshek's physical needs the first morning, I invited him to tell me something about himself. He said, "I am a Jew, what more is there to tell." My only knowledge of Jews was what I had learned in Bible class and Toshek did not appear to be, or to live, like those people, and so Toshek's reply did not give me any insight. As the days passed, however, we began to communicate more freely and I could sense that he was also curious about me.

Toshek's wife, Malva, was a pleasant lady who talked freely from the beginning and so I gained from her some essential understanding of Toshek as a person. She also began talking about Jewish culture by explaining the values and attitudes which influenced Jewish thought. Jews, she said, had a great reverence for life and therefore with how life was used, and this extended to a reverence for people. Learning, she told me, had always had a central place in Jewish culture, especially Talmudic (religious) learning. The man of learning was treasured above all others and referred to as one of the "beautiful people."[13] The concept of the family is extremely important in the Jewish culture. In addition, industriousness and material success were considered important but always secondary to learning. Material success was perceived as a *mitsva* (blessing from God). Malva told me that even well-educated Jewish women remain in an inferior position to men. The traditional Jewish man thanks God daily for the fact that he was not born a woman. Males have a social, economic, and political status over women in the traditional Jewish culture. Knowledge of these basic cultural values became of great importance to me in clarifying and maintaining a favorable family-nurse interaction. Evaluation of my performance depended on understanding and relating to these values.

The average Belgian Jew in 1958 had a poor concept of a nurse because the nurse's role was perceived to be subservient, and the nurse a person of minimal intelligence who relied heavily on the physician for direction. Scottish nursing education did not develop this type of nurse, and so I was a puzzle to Toshek. While I attended his needs with regularity I did not perceive myself in the role of serving wench. Instead, to Toshek I displayed an alarming intelligence and made independent decisions about his care based on my own nursing values and observations. He was amazed to discover this behavior and that I also understood political and economic world affairs plus literature and music. So it was a cultural shock to his perception of a nurse and a woman.

RECIPROCAL CONFUSION

Shortly after my arrival in Toshek's home I perceived the importance of the family. Within a few days I was convinced that I was being spied upon by members of the extended family as they came to meet Toshek's nurse. It seemed there was never a minute when I was not being observed by one of the family members. I did not know that what I was experiencing was a cultural behavior pattern highly acceptable to a kin-based family. After an initial perplexed and slightly angry period, I asked Malva whether I was distrusted. She looked very embarrassed and asked what had given me such a strange idea. When I told her what was worrying me, she laughed and explained that traditional Jewish people believe that the act of charity performed by visiting a sick person mitigates his illness.

Every evening at about five o'clock (earlier on Fridays because Sabbath was about to begin) a handsome white-haired gentleman would come to visit the patient. He was a quiet and solemn man whom I often heard softly humming. He was introduced to me as Toshek's elder brother and was acknowledged as the head of the family, the patriarch, a deeply religious man. (I later discovered that his humming was praying.)

LEARNING MORE ABOUT THE PATIENT'S CULTURE

Most of my time was spent taking care of Toshek's needs, and I found he was a humble, friendly person despite his wealth. When he felt well enough he would listen to music or read books written in a strange script which I thought was Arabic but was in fact Yiddish, the language of the Shtetl communities, which is written in Hebrew characters. (Weinrich[13] has written an interesting article on this language which might be of further interest to some readers.) At times I enjoyed Toshek but often I felt inadequate to meet his complex emotional, spiritual, and intellectual needs. My abilities to comprehend or deal with these complex needs seemed meager, and I found myself limiting the time I spent with the patient in these early days.

Sometimes Toshek wept in self-pity or railed in anger at his fate. He denounced the eminent cardiologist who took care of him. He accused the family of neglecting him and yet they seemed almost overly attentive to him. Although we all cared for him, none could change his fate. I became more frustrated daily with my inability to help Toshek. My Christian background had taught me abnegation and resignation, but attempts to help Toshek accept his illness by explaining and using such concepts were rejected. The words which were appropriate to Christians and made sense in the light of my value system failed miserably. It is difficult to comfort a Jew by citing Christ as an example of patient acceptance. I tried to evaluate his needs from a Jewish viewpoint but was unable to achieve this goal. It was then I began to see clearly the important part culture plays in our life expectations and reactions to life's demands upon us.

Toshek's family belonged to a group of Jews who called themselves "modern traditional" since the second World War. Within this group traditions of culture are observed such as separation of meat and milk foods, including dishes and cooking utensils (kosher), and observation of religious ceremonies on Fridays, Saturdays, and special feast days. Food is prepared in advance of all holy days and only a minimal amount of necessary work is done on those days. Those who are deeply religious do not light fire nor use it on holy days. Most of the people in this group do not ride in trains or automobiles on holy days of religious observance. The men attend the synagogue accompanied by their sons. Women occasionally attend the synagogue, walking to and from it in the company of their female children. Men and women sit in separate areas in the synagogue according to the old tradition. Marriage ceremonies are observed in the traditional fashion with the bride preparing herself for marriage by taking ritual baths at the synagogue. A bridal contract is made in the presence of family members and the rabbi. The marriage takes place under a canopy in the synagogue, with the rabbi and cantor. Traditional family blessings are prayed over the young couple by the most revered family members. Traditional Jewish dances are still performed at the reception.

As Toshek's family observed and followed their traditions, I learned much about their rich cultural heritage. More and more I realized that lack of knowledge about Jewish culture limited the quality of health care I might provide, and so I made a formal request to the family to be instructed about their culture. The family was quick to respond for they too had a high regard for learning and they planned ways to help me learn. There is a strong oral tradition among Jewish people, and Toshek was a born story-teller. When he was feeling well enough, he would talk of Jewish history and explain their religion and ritual. We listened together to the great traditional cantors on records, and he explained the prayers and taught me to appreciate the free expression in the music. He also taught me modern

Jewish history, culminating in suspense stories of the war years and the time he spent in hiding with the Maquis (the French underground army).

Edith, his daughter, became a friend as she shared her books with me and explained the trends of modern Jewish thought. I became familiar with Jewish literature and read avidly the lives of Jabotinsky and Herzl, the giants and founding fathers of Israelian Zionism. Edith talked with me about contemporary Jewish problems in the areas of language and culture and occasionally shared with me her personal hopes and dreams.

Toshek's wife, Malva, who was keenly intellectual, explored with me the movement of European Jewry toward integration with the dominant culture stream prior to World War II. Particularly in Germany, Austria, France, Belgium, and Holland, many Jewish young people had chosen to integrate into the mainstream culture rather than embrace the ideals of Zionism. When Hitler's regime expanded to the development of a pure Aryan race, it became evident that the Jewish cultural heritage formed a barrier to integration. The family told me that a new wave of dedication to cultural and traditional practices occurred, in some cases with a deep religious component, and in others with simply a strong revival of traditional practice divorced from the religious component. This idea was difficult for me to comprehend since Jewish tradition has a religious base.

Malva also talked with me about Jewish political affiliations. We discussed music, art, and literature along with the problems and achievements of Jewish women. In time, Malva and I came to know each other well as she saw me trying to meet Toshek's needs. This helped her develop a trusting relationship with me. It seemed that each member of the extended family took an interest in helping me become acculturated. I learned much about Jewish culture including the dietary laws and their relationship to the patient's peace of mind. I took part in religious feasts and family festivals, and when the time came, I helped to prepare a clean passover (Kosher Pesakh). Indeed, I began to feel that I had been accorded a place in the family. If I were asked if it was necessary to become an integral part of another person's culture to fulfill a helping role, I would answer in the negative. From my experiences, it does not seem necessary (or even desirable) to "go native" in order to demonstrate one's willingness to accept another patient's cultural values, norms, and practices as part of his lifestyle. I believe it is necessary, however, to protect the patient's right in order to fulfill his important cultural obligations.

DEVELOPING NEW NURSING SKILLS

The nursing care required by Toshek was of course my central focus. He could be very demanding and challenged the effectiveness of traditional nursing care practices. In the beginning, Toshek showed anxiety and doubt as his cultural perceptions of my nurse's role conflicted with the behaviors he observed in me. Initially, when I made decisions about his care or management, he thought this was the prerogative of the physician, and he would become anxious or insist on Malva calling the cardiologist. When this had occurred on several occasions, the physician merely confirmed my decisions and Toshek ceased to be fearful.

Toshek was often very emotional. As I learned more about his culture I interpreted his behavior differently and began to see cultural significance in it. I perceived that at times his pain was not physical but rather emotional anguish arising from present and past life experiences. Sometimes it seemed to be the echo of a cry for help arising from the Jewish people, a cry which had gone unanswered in history. Sometimes his anger was not directed toward me but toward those other people who had unleashed pogroms on his ancestors or taken his family to the gas chambers. At other times, Toshek's frustrations were real and directed towards me. He would shake his head and say, "strange non-Jewish woman" (*Vreemd goyish meidl*). I understood his feelings and the conflict within him. It was unusual for a Jewish man to trust a non-Jewish woman, especially after the terrors of the war years. He also found it frightening to admit that he felt affection for me. His behavior placed real demands upon me but, as my knowledge of his culture increased, I found myself willing to risk the therapeutic use of myself.

In time, I could distinguish between physical pain and anguish. Toshek called both states pain. It was possible for me to test his phenomena as his physical pain was often greatly relieved, whereas his anguish could not be relieved effectively by medicine. In such moments I would listen and empathize with Toshek, and his anxiety would subside. There was no need for me to dissimulate interest, because I cared about the welfare of the patient. I was moved by the history of his people and their agonies and impressed with their rich culture.

I came to realize that in a kin-based society, the children in the family play an important role, and sometimes a small service offered Toshek by a child of the family was more helpful than my professional care. I learned to channel care through the family to him, providing extra satisfactions for him. One of the happiest moments he experienced was when he learned that his daughter was pregnant. He said, "Now I can die in peace."

As the months passed, evidences that I was accepted and trusted became more frequent. For example, when decisions were made by the family which affected Toshek, I was included in the family conference. Again, when Toshek's condition deteriorated, the head of the family asked my advice about calling a consultant, and an eminent specialist from France was flown in by helicopter. Additional evidence was the growing extent of my influence within the extended family in that Malva and Edith talked about their conflicts regarding Toshek's condition with me. Other members of the family asked me to help solve their marital problems; I worked with a teenager who was having psychosocial problems and made suggestions about the management of the youngest member of the family, a child only a few weeks old.

RESOLUTION

As Toshek became gravely ill, the family realized his approaching death, and I was integrated into the family. The men of the family would talk with me about management of Toshek and accepted the suggestions I made for his comfort. Although two other nurses were brought into the situation to assist with the care of Toshek, no decisions were made for him without consulting me. When Toshek became acutely ill for the last time, the cardiologist decided to hospitalize him. This happened on a Friday evening, the beginning of the Jewish Sabbath. I was not with him then, but he was transported to the hospital accompanied by six adult members of the family. He kept asking for me, and the family searched in the city until they found me. When I reached the hospital, it was nearly sundown and Toshek greeted me with the traditional *Shabbas* (which loosely translates, "We will celebrate this day together.") He had never before greeted me with this traditional greeting used among Eastern European Jews. He asked the time and when I told him, he sent all the members of the family home to prepare for Sabbath. This was a significant act with reference to the nurse-patient relationship. To choose to stay alone with me on the holy day of the week indicated, again, that I was part of the family.

As the therapeutic process had developed, Toshek was occasionally able to speak of death in an abstract way with reference to others but seldom at this time of his own death. Later, however, he explained the traditional dying practices of the Jews in the Shtetl communities and asked whether I would arrange for him to die in the traditional manner, namely, lying on the floor, covered but naked. Because I expected Toshek to die in his own home I made a solemn promise to fulfill his wish. On the evening before his death he reminded me of this promise.

Within the nurse-patient relationship, I experienced a deep inner conflict between my own Scottish cultural values, the subcultural values of the nursing profession, and my desire to respect the patient's traditional values. It seemed cruel to have Toshek die on a hard terrazzo floor and the subcultural values of nursing had imbued me with a desire to nurture and support dying people with physical comfort measures. Nonetheless, Toshek's cultural and religious values dictated that he should return to God as he was born, without the embellishments of the world. Part of my conflict lay in the judgment which I could expect from physicians and associates as I was certain that they would misinterpret my intentions and label the incident "bizarre." I worried about the fuss which I could anticipate from the hospital administrators. When the cardiologist and a group of consultants came to make their morning visit, I told them of the patient's desire. Some were appalled and others were so uncomfortable at the thought that they giggled. One house physician returned after the others left and said that if I called him when death seemed imminent he would help me put Toshek on the floor. Several members of the family were present when I decided he was close to death and with the help of the physician we laid him on the floor. Toshek had come to trust me and I felt a moment of great sadness when he could not respond to me when I asked if he knew I had kept my promise.

I had been Toshek's day nurse for a year and seven months at the time of his death. I grieved with the family. We departed from the hospital promptly leaving his body with four male family members who remained and prayed throughout the day. According to Jewish law, his body could not be moved until after sundown. His body was brought to his home in a sealed casket before the burial. Women do not go to the burial. Malva had a family member call and ask me to come and take part in the ritual mourning with her, to keep Shiveh in the idiom of the Shtetl. I was deeply moved by the request. It is very unusual for a stranger to be invited to keep Shiveh and almost unknown if the person is a Christian. Malva sat barefooted on a low stool, wearing a shredded garment (the sign of widowhood). The men of the family did not shave for at least a month after Toshek's death, indicating their dissociation from worldly things during the initial time of mourning.

Recapping the Nurse-Patient Relationship Phases and Themes

During the initiation phase of any nurse-patient relationship several main themes occur: (1) mutual sharing of knowledge about each other and the situation, (2) testing of the nurse by the patient, and (3) the emergence of a helping modality. In a transcultural situation, the first theme takes a longer period than in a situation between a nurse and patient of the same cultural background. This phase of initiation is one of great importance in all therapeutic relationships but particularly in a transcultural setting. Leininger has said, "The scientific and humanistic integration of culture into health practices is a relatively new undertaking for health practitioners. It is, however, an extremely important part of providing for optimal care to patients."[3] The nurse must, therefore, develop a cultural awareness. It is not realistic to expect a patient to divorce himself from his cultural background and to react in accordance with the norms of the dominant culture simply because he finds himself in the midst of the dominant culture. Instead, it is more reasonable to expect the nurse to learn to understand cultural differences in order to deliver optimal care. Nurses often label patients in transcultural situations as difficult, stubborn, strange, or impossible when, in fact, the patient is simply being himself, a person based on a tradition often not known or understood by the practitioner.

The discomfort which I felt in the early stages of the relationship had to do with my lack of knowledge of the patient and his culture. Toshek tested me on many occasions. He would tease me saying, "The British are shocked at everything," which I read as an attempt to make me retort unfavorably about Jewish culture. He would, also, tell stories of the inefficiency and lack of personal cleanliness he had observed in French nurses, an attempt to test me professionally. This was, also, the period during which he doubted my ability to diagnose his physiological problems, another lack of trust or testing situation.

During this initial phase of the nurse-patient relationship, it is necessary for the nurse to gain knowledge which will enable her to understand the patient by putting herself in his place. The helping process cannot be established until the nurse understands the patient's needs. Before reaching this understanding the nurse is no more than a general administrator of care. After this understanding is reached, the nurse becomes an essential part of the therapeutic process. In order to empathize with a patient, the nurse must understand his background. Travelbee says, "The ability to predict behavior or comprehend the behavior of another is limited by personal background,"[11] and "empathetic boundaries may be expanded by repeated contacts with individuals of varying backgrounds."[12] Mere contact is not enough, however. Without a realization that cultural values, attitudes, beliefs, and life styles vary and a willingness to explore the situation from the patient's place in the scheme, a therapeutic relationship is difficult to develop. Empathy cannot be achieved without understanding, which presupposes a knowledge of the patient's basic values. Glittenberg says, "Reading someone from another culture mandates understanding and acceptance of his way of thinking."[1] Therapeutic use of self is not without risk. The nurse, and especially the student, is open to possible discomfort in the interaction process, unless she is equipped with the appropriate cultural knowledge on which to build the nurse-patient relationship and develop it beyond the administrative phase. Therapeutic use of self is the ultimate in nursing process for the nurse who desires to assist the patient to find meaning in illness.

THERAPEUTIC MANEUVERS

During the continuation phase of the nurse-patient relationship many therapeutic maneuvers were employed in our attempt to help the patient uncover and deal with his feelings and eventually to find some meaning in his illness. Toshek was encouraged to express his feelings, and to cope with the hostilites he felt toward the world, his family, and fate. Occasionally, it was necessary to help him develop self-limiting techniques when his behavior caused his wife undue stress. After the therapeutic relationship had been entered into, I attempted to provide support for him in his depressed and anguished moments. One of the maneuvers which in retrospect I see as valuable to the patient was encouraging him to speak, when he wished, of his childhood. It seemed to me that in reviewing his entire life and expressing its satisfactions audibly he was better able to contemplate his approaching death. It was also during such sessions that I came to know much about the culture of the Shtetl communities.

EVALUATION MODALITIES

Hofling, Leininger and Bregg state: "Bringing a nurse-patient relationship to a close is as important as getting the relationship into action," but that "what actually occurs when the relationship between the nurse and the patient draws to a close is not so well-known, as the other previously discussed phases of the nurse-patient relationship."[2] Closure of nurse-patient relationships are certainly important. A therapeutic relationship is usually concluded by the patient leaving the hospital, the judging that the time is ripe, or determining if the personal commitment of the nurse to the patient is causing too much discomfort. How closure is achieved in many nurse-patient relationships is not known. Traditionally, the nurse has been charged with the task of developing a state of uninvolved involvement, a state which is a contradiction in terms and is particularly difficult in transcultural situations. It is difficult to pursue such an "uninvolved" relationship while learning to appreciate a new culture. This is even more difficult for the nurse in a transcultural situation as the nurse must be willing to risk herself therapeutically if she is to gain credence. Some degree of personal involvement is unavoidable and essential.

Nurses engaged in psychotherapeutic relationships have been taught the dangers of continued interaction with the patient beyond a certain period of need. Some colleges of nursing teach the psychotherapeutic process with explicit criteria for the closure of relationships. I believe the establishment of explicit criteria for the closing of nurse-patient relationships could result in restrained relationships and patient doubt as to the authenticity of the nurse's caring attitude. In the case cited, criteria were based upon the health of the patient, and the relationship was continued beyond the usual period of time. The criteria used were (1) the desire of the patient or family for such continued interaction, and (2) recognition of a changing focus in the relationship. Thus I have continued my interaction with the family for fifteen years.

Immediately after the death of the patient, I continued in a therapeutic role with the family members as they worked their way through the grief process. The contacts became fewer and fewer, and the focus of the relationship changed many times in the course of past years. Presently, the contacts are limited to occasional letters and phone calls. I evaluate, however, the continuation of interest in the family's well-being as a realistic result of affective and effective earlier nurse-patient-family exchanges. Although, the nurse-patient relationship is essentially based on patient need, it is not possible to live through a deep human experience such as we do with some patients and their families and forget them. We as nurses also change our feelings and skills. We learn in each encounter something new about ourselves and are assisted in our "becoming."[10]

Rogers[8] in explicating patient-centered therapy has indicated that he has continued contact with clients for many years. To risk oneself in a transcultural nursing situation and in a therapeutic role is something bewildering (even a little scary), but it is only in an atmosphere of genuine caring that the patient (especially the patient with terminal illness) can find some meaning in illness. I am confirmed in my thinking by the words of Rogers to a client, "All I know is what I am feeling and that is, I feel very close to you at the moment." This is a statement of genuine caring on the part of the therapeutic figure.

Conclusion

Returning at this point to Leininger's question as to whether one can become a helping person in a kin-based society other than one's own culture, I would answer in the affirmative. A skillful nurse willing to learn about a culture new to her and to risk herself in new kinds of nurse-patient relationships can fill such a role.

The nursing profession in the United States could be viewed as standing at the most exciting point in its entire history. The equal rights amendment to the Constitution and the impetus given to women's rights by the Women's Movement are creating opportunities for nurses to be heard. The traditional position of handmaiden has been rejected, and the nurse, male or female, is articulating freely about the profession and its goals.

Nurses are developing a body of knowledge which is peculiarly their own and impressing the public with their educational accomplishments. Innovative nursing practice legislation makes it possible for American nurses to practice legally roles which have been theirs for decades. An autonomy that has been surreptitious in the past has come into the open. Consequently, the nurse has a greater responsibility for the quality of care offered to patients and an increasing obligation to listen to consumer demands and serve as consumer advocates. We are at last free to make decisions about our professional needs in education, education which should equip us to deliver health care at a level of competence and relevance hitherto unknown.

Members of minority cultures across the country are demanding health care which meets their cultural needs, and since we are now free to plan health education curricula as we see fit, let us include the long neglected dimension of culture. Currently, there are a few nursing schools giving serious consideration to cultural deficits in the curricula. A very few have included basic cultural anthropology as an early prerequisite to the nursing major. Some schools are beginning to consider the development of undergraduate and graduate courses on the subject of transcultural nursing.

In this article I have tried to demonstrate that knowledge of cultural background, values, and attitudes of the patient are indispensible for nurses who wish to deliver comprehensive health care. Total care can become a reality only when patients are seen in the framework of their individual cultural patterns.

FOOTNOTES

1. Glittenberg, J.: Adapting health care to a cultural setting. American Journal of Nursing 74:2219-2220, December 1974
2. Hofling, C. K.; Leininger, M., and Bregg, E.: Basic Psychiatric Concepts in Nursing. J. P. Lippincott, Philadelphia, 1967, p. 66.

3. Leininger, M.: Nursing and Anthropology: Two Worlds to Blend. John Wiley and Sons, New York, 1970, pp. 29-30.
4. Ibid., p. 45.
5. Leininger, M.: Using cultural styles in the helping process and in relation to the subculture of nursing. Nursing Papers. State of Illinois, Chicago, 1972, p. 43.
6. Leininger, M.: Transcultural Nursing: Theory and Practice. John Wiley and Sons, New York, In press.
7. Osborne, O. H.: Anthropology and nursing: some common traditions and interests. Nursing Research 18:251, 1969.
8. Rogers, C. R.: Meador and Rogers. Client Centered Therapy. Current Psychotherapies. Raymond Corsini (Ed.). F. E. Peacock Publishing, Inc., New York, 1973, pp. 162-163.
9. Rogers, C. R.: "A theory of therapy, personality, and interpersonal relationships as developed in the client-centered framework," in Psychology: A Study of a Science, Vo. III, Formulations of the Person and the Social Context. McGraw-Hill Book Company, New York, 1959, pp. 84-156.
10. Rogers, C.: On Becoming a Person. Houghton Mifflin Company, Boston, 1961.
11. Travelbee, J.: Interpersonal Aspects of Nursing. F.A. Davis Company, Philadelphia, 1966, pp. 16-19.
12. Ibid, p. 203.
13. Weinrich, M.: Yiddishkayt and yiddish, in Mordicai M. Kaplan Jubilee Volume. Jewish Theological Seminary of America, New York, 1953.
14. Zbrowoski, M. and Hertzog, E.: Life is with People. Shocken Books, New York, 1952.

Illness and Indignity*

Thomas S. Szasz

All of us in the health professions share certain fundamental aspirations and goals, among which the most important ones are keeping the healthy person healthy; restoring the sick person to health; and, most generally, safeguarding and prolonging life. That these ends are so overwhelming good and noble is what makes their pursuit so gratifying, and those in the health professions so richly honored and rewarded.

Life would be simpler than it is if health and longevity were its only, or even its principal, purposes; or, to put it differently, if there were no goals or values that often conflict with their pursuit. One of the values that men and women — and children, too — cherish, and that often conflicts with their pursuit of health at any cost, is dignity.

Dignity is, of course, that ineffable and yet obvious quality of human encounters and situations that enriches the participants' self-esteem. For example, in these ceremonies we, your elders and teachers, dignify you the graduates, and you, in turn, dignify us. This process of dignification is characteristically mutual or reciprocal. Dignified conduct in one person or party generates dignified conduct in another, and vice versa.

Conversely, indignity is that equally obvious, but much more easily definable quality of human encounters and situations, that impoverishes the participants' self-esteem. There are many forms and types of it, and one of the most common and most tragic is the indignity of disability, illness, and old age. Many sick persons behave, simply because of their illness, in ways that make their conduct — on the face of it and by definition — undignified. When a person loses control over his basic bodily functions, when he cannot control his speech or skeletal musculature, when he cannot work, then — often against his most intense efforts — he is rendered, undignified. Language, the oldest but still the most reliable guide to a people's true sentiments, starkly reveals this intimate connection between illness and indignity. In English, we use the same word to describe an expired or otherwise worthless passport or ticket, an indefensible argument, an illegitimate legal document or contract, and a person disabled by disease. We call each of them "invalid." To be an invalid, then, is to be an invalidated person, a human being stamped "not valid" by the invisible but invincible hand of popular opinion. While invalidism carries with it the heaviest burden of indignity, some of this stigma adheres to virtually all illness, to virtually any participation in the patient role.

From *The Journal of the American Medical Association*, Vol. 227, No. 5,
pp. 543-545, February 4, 1974. Copyright 1974, American Medical Association.
By the permission of the author and publisher.
*Read in part as the commencement address before the College of Health
Related Professions, State University of New York, Upstate Medical Center,
Syracuse, New York, June 3, 1973.

This fact generates two very important problems for persons in the health professions: one is that the sick person's undignified behavior may stimulate or release the professional person's inclination to respond with undignified behavior of his own; the other is that patients disabled in ways that render them grossly undignified may prefer death with dignity to life without it. Let me offer a few observations on each of these.

The Indignity of Being a Patient

The connections between illness and indignity are, in the main, quite obvious. Because the patient cannot work, cannot take care of himself, must disrobe and submit his body for examination by strangers — for these and many other equally good reasons, the sick person perceives himself as suffering not only from an illness but also from a loss of dignity. Moreover, the patient's loss of dignity often generates a reciprocal loss of respect for him by those around him, especially by his family and physicians. This unfortunate process of degradation is often concealed, though in my opinion never very successfully, by the imagery and vocabulary of paternalism — family and physician treating the patient as if he were a child (or child-like), and the patient treating them as if they were his parents (or superiors).

This fundamental tendency — to "infantilize" the sick person and to "parentify" the healer — manifests itself in countless ways in the everyday practice of medicine. For example, the patient is expected to trust his physician, but the physician need not trust his patient; the patient is expected to impart his intimate bodily and personal experiences to the physician, while the physician may withhold vital information from the patient.

The patient's undignified position vis-à-vis the medical authorities is symbolized by the linguistic structure of the medical situation: the sick person speaks, as it were, only one language, while the healer speaks two. The patient communicates in ordinary language, which he shares with his physician; the physician communicates partly in the same language, insofar as he speaks *to* his patient, and partly in another language, insofar as he speaks *about* him. The physician's second language used to be Latin, and now is the technical idiom or jargon of medicine. The upshot is that patients often do not know or understand what is wrong with them, what is in their medical records, or what drugs they are taking. To be sure, like children or other fearful, humiliated, or oppressed persons, patients often do not want to know these things. Yet even if this were so — and of course, it is not always so — it would not, in my opinion, justify withholding such information from them. After all, many people do not want to know what is under the hood of an automobile, but we would not accept this as justifying automobile manufacturers in maintaining a systematic policy of withholding this information from car buyers or releasing it to them only under special circumstances.

My point is that many people today accept it as right and proper that patients should not understand the prescriptions their physician hands them or that they should not know what is in their hospital records; at the same time, they object to the indignities which the medical situation often imposes on them. The result of this ambivalence and inarticulated conflict is that people often feel anxious and humiliated at the prospect of seeking medical care and frequently avoid or reject such care altogether.

In other words, we must keep in mind that people want and need not only health but also dignity, that often they can obtain health only at the cost of dignity, and that sometimes they prefer not to pay this price. The evidence for this view is so obvious that we may fail to notice it on that very account. It is obvious, for example, that patients participate most eagerly and most intelligently in medical situations that entail little or no humiliation on their part. Thus, people seek help freely for refractive errors of their eyes or for athletic injuries. On the other hand, it is equally obvious that patients participate most reluctantly or not at all in those medical situations that entail a great deal of humiliation on their part. Thus, people are much more reluctant to seek medical help for syphilis or gonorrhea — even though these diseases can now be treated effectively and safely! — then they do for astigmatism or presbyopia. Often, they do not seek medical help at all for those conditions whose treatment is humiliating to the point of legally articulated stigmatization, such as drug addiction or the so-called psychoses.

There is, I submit, a practical lesson in this for all of us: namely, that it is not enough that we in the health professions do a technically competent job of healing the patient's body; we must do an equally competent job of safeguarding his dignity and self-esteem. In proportion as we fail in this latter task, we forfeit — indeed, we destroy — the practical value of our technical competence for the sick person.

The Conflict Between Protecting Health and Protecting Dignity

I have suggested, and we know only too well, that efforts to regain health or prolong life often conflict with the need to maintain dignity. Thus arises a moral dilemma of quite general, perhaps even universal, dimensions. In this connection, I find the currently popular phrase "death with dignity" quite misleading; it isn't so much that people want to die with dignity, but rather that they want to live with it. The phrase is symptomatic of some of our contemporary moral predicaments. It is precisely because so many persons now live without dignity that they also die without it. Active and dignified persons, whether soldiers or surgeons, have always wanted to die with their boots on. Military men have traditionally preferred death on the battlefield or even suicide to surrender and loss of face; medical men prefer a sudden death from a myocardial infarct to a lingering demise from generalized carcinomatosis. I cite these examples only to support my suggestion that there is often an irreconcilable antagonism between preserving and promoting dignity and preserving and promoting health.

There are, of course, many such antagonisms in life, which is what makes human existence tragic in the classical Greek and Christian conceptions of it. For example, in personal and political affairs, we desire both freedom and security, but can often gain the one only at the expense of the other. The modern scientific and technical outlook, valuable though it is for realizing scientific and technical ends, misleads us badly insofar as it deals in isolation, as it were, with the concepts of health and dignity and promises to maximize each at the cost of nothing more than scientific and technical effort and know-how. This perspective has led to a lopsided and, indeed, quite erroneous estimate of the bargain or trade-off entailed in maintaining or securing good health. I refer to the now widely held view that people can become progressively healthier as a result of scientific advances — fashionably called "breakthroughs" — in medicine, without individual persons having to make any sacrifices for it; that is, without their having to pay for it, without their having to curb their appetites and passions, and without their having to suffer some loss of dignity. The result is that an immense amount of contemporary illness is directly or indirectly self-induced, through things people ingest or inject that they should not, or fail to ingest or inject that they should.

Is Health Worth the Price of Dignity?

The irreconcilable conflict that may arise between prolonging life and maintaining dignity was, as were all the fundamental conflicts characteristic of the human condition, well appreciated and articulated by the ancient Greeks. In the "Phaedo," Plato illustrates this dilemma and Socrates' method of resolving it.

The "Death Scene" opens with Socrates and some of his closest friends gathered in anticipation of Socrates drinking the hemlock. After some conversation between Socrates and his friends, Socrates says farewell and asks the executioner to bring the poisoned cup. But Crito urges Socrates to wait, to prolong his life for as long as he may: "But Socrates," he pleads, "I know that other men take the poison quite late, and eat and drink heartily, and even enjoy the company of their chosen friends, after the announcement has been made. So do not hurry; there is still time."

Socrates' reply articulates the distinction between life as a biological process that may and perhaps ought to be prolonged for as long as possible, and as a spiritual pilgrimage that can and should be traversed and ended in a proper manner. This is what Socrates says:

> And those whom you speak of, Crito, naturally do so; for they think that they will be the gainers by so doing. And I naturally shall not do so; for I think that I should gain nothing by drinking the poison a little later but my own contempt for so greedily saving up a life which is already spent.

The distinction between the death of the body and the end of life, which is the difference between Crito's and Socrates' outlook on life and death, continues to baffle us in the health sciences. The main reason why this is the case is, remarkably, also explained by Socrates.

Crito asks his friend how he wants to be buried. Socrates replies:

> Crito thinks that I am the body which he will presently see as a corpse, and he asks me how he is to bury me. All the arguments which I have used to prove that I shall not remain with you after I have drunk the poison . . . have been thrown away on him. . . . For, dear Crito, you must know that to use words wrongly is not only a fault in itself, it also corrupts the soul. You must be of good cheer, and say that you are burying my body; and you may bury it as you please, and you think right.

The distinction Socrates makes here between himself and his body is at once obvious and elusive; you know as well as I do how often modern people — scientifically informed and enlightened people — fail to make this distinction.

The richness of "The Death Scene" for our theme is by no means exhausted by my foregoing remarks on it. There is significance, too, in Socrates' parting words. "Crito," he says, "I owe a cock to Asclepius; do not forget it."

The ritual sacrifice Socrates here requests his friend to make on his behalf refers to the custom of offering, on recovering from sickness, a cock to Asclepius, the god of healing. In other words, Socrates viewed his death as a recovery from an illness, presaging the Christian view of it.

In short, the message I have wanted to bring to you is simply this: Do your utmost to exercise your skills in healing, but do not do so by sacrificing dignity, either your patient's or your own — these two being tied together by bonds not unlike those of matrimony, except, especially in these days, stronger. For, if I may paraphrase the Scriptures, what does it profit a man if he gains his health but loses his dignity?

The Patient-Client as a Consumer: Some Observations on the Changing Professional-Client Relationship

Leo G. Reeder

Sociologists have had a long-standing concern with professional-client relations, particularly the doctor-patient relationship (Freidson, 1961; Bloom, 1963; Wilson, 1963; Scott and Volkart, 1966; Mechanic, 1968). In most of this literature the discussion concerns the client's role in the medical care system in terms of "patient behavior"; the role of the client is seen as a major contingency in the structure of medical care. More recently, Wilson and Bloom (1972) have examined the Parsonian model of the doctor-patient relationship and have presented alternative models that amplify and change the role analysis of patient-practitioner relationships. "The patient is assumed to take a passively dependent posture in many if not most health-care interaction . . ." (Bloom and Wilson, 1972). Reviewing this role-set very briefly, we note that as a distinctive type of occupation, professions have been successful in obtaining institutional powers that set limits on client freedoms and powers. Professional expertise becomes institutionalized in a form similar to bureaucratic office (Freidson, 1970c).

In capsule form, the features of professionalism include: autonomy, protection from encroachment, control of production and application of knowledge, and a code of ethics. The client as a patient may be treated as an object; he may receive little information concerning the treatment processes and the possible outcomes. The professional's conception of his relation to his client determines such communicative failures. Medical "orders" determine the entire gamut of activities involving patient care.

When seeking information, the patient is often told by ancillary personnel, "Sorry, you'll have to ask the doctor"; but when asked, the physician is typically disinclined to provide information to the patient. Even when communication is deliberate, as in prescribing a treatment regimen, any breakdown in communication is attributed to the culpability of the patient. Giving information to the client-patient becomes a "management problem" for the physician. There is insistence on faith or trust in the professional client-patient relationship thus neutralizing threatened or demeaned status in the layman's requests for explanation and justification (Freidson, 1970c).

Recently, social structural changes occurring in the health care field indicate that the relationships of professional-client are undergoing a radical process of change. Some critics have observed that the present

From *Journal of Health & Social Behaviour*, Vol. 13, No. 4, December 1972. By permission of the author and publisher.

system of health services is marked by a "professional decision-making apparatus — whose values and priorities may not reflect society's goals" (Levin, 1969). Others state that

> There is no proper surrogate, no substitute for the direct expression of his interest and needs by the patient himself . . . (a reorganized system of medical care) establishes the essential right, indeed obligation, of the patient to serve as an active participant in the process of shaping the services that are supposed to exist for his benefit (Freidson, 1970b).

In bureaucratic settings, professional autonomy may be modified by organizational imperatives. But the professional may use the established structure for his own ends to "control the circumstances under which service is given" (Haug and Sussman, 1969). Simultaneously, the client of professional services in such settings tends to redefine the situation so that he is viewed as a consumer. In the public school sector, for example, the client is making strenuous efforts to obtain a greater degree of control over the services provided by the professional educational establishment. Parents press the system to obtain local control over curriculum, employment, tenure, and other fundamental policies long thought to be the sole prerogative of the professional. It appears that the clients are in revolt against the practitioner's work autonomy and it is a group rather than a personal rejection phenomenon.

This paper addresses itself to the implications for changes in the traditional professional-client relationship in health care consequent to changes in the structure of medical care. The changes we refer to relate to the following: (1) orientation of medical care away from "treatment" to "prevention"; (2) provision of medical services within bureaucratic structures, as distinct from the solo practice of medicine, and the growing sophistication with bureaucracy; and (3) the growth of consumerism as a social movement. The analysis will draw upon the conceptual framework of both professionalism and social movements, and the implications for changes in the professional-client relationship.

Structural Changes In Society Related to Health Care

One of the most significant changes that has occurred in the developed societies has been a shift in medical care from curative to preventive types of services. This is not to say that curative medicine is no longer an important feature of medical care; rather, the focus of attention has shifted significantly toward the prevention of chronic diseases as the control of acute and/or infectious diseases has been accomplished. In a system dominated by curative or emergency care there is a "seller's market." The customer is suspect; client-professional relationships tend to be characterized by the traditional mode of interaction so well described in the literature. On the other hand, when prevention of illness is emphasized, the client has to be persuaded that he has a need for medical services such as periodic check-ups. The person has to be encouraged to come into the physician's office for medical care. Under these circumstances, there are elements of a "buyer's market"; in such situations there is more tendency for the "customers to be right." Theoretically, at least, this is the posture taken by the seller or provider of services.

A second feature of societal change concerns the growing sophistication with bureaucracy. In the health care field there has been a considerable development of prepaid health care programs organized by private practitioners and others. This development will undoubtedly be accelerated by the federally-encouraged Health Maintenance Organizations. Thus, increasingly, non-welfare, paying patients will receive medical care in some type of organizational milieu. Partly, this is related to the fact that, as society becomes more urbanized and industrialized, large-scale bureaucratic institutions commonly associated with this phenomenon become a pervasive feature of society. Sociologists have recognized that certain norms, i.e., dress, time, order and authority, are rather rigorously prescribed by these institutions. Furthermore, Inkeles has shown that the distinctive roles engendered by the industrial system:

> ... also foster typical patterns of perception, opinions, beliefs, and values which are not institutionally prescribed but arise spontaneously as new subcultures in response to the institutional conditions provided by the typically differentiated role-structure of modern industrial society (Inkeles, 1960).

Thus, individual and collective social perception, and action tend to be influenced by the patterning of the industrial or other large-scale institutions. The paper by Inkeles demonstrates that large-scale bureaucratic industrial systems tend to generate similar types of responses by people in different countries. Using this same theoretical approach, it can be assumed that within a given industrialized society the process would obtain for a variety of standard environments with standard institutional pressures for particular groups. Hence, to the degree that this obtains, relatively standard patterns of experience, attitudes, and value pressures should be produced (Inkeles, 1960). We suggest that similar institutional arrangements in the health-care field would result in processes similar to those described by Inkeles. The result would be a "shared perspective" on the part of individuals and collectivities that is significant for the growth of the consumerism phenomenon as a social movement, particularly in the health field as discussed below. The bureaucratic features of the profession of medicine plus the increasing bureaucratization of delivery of personal health services combine to create institutionalized, more or less standardized, environments that provide standard patterns of experience, attitudes, and values to the participants in the system, providers and consumers alike.

The third feature of societal change to be noted is the development of consumerism. During the decade of the sixties a new concept came into prominence in the delivery of health services in this country. This was the concept of the person as a *consumer* rather than as a patient (Bashshur, 1967; Hochbaum, 1969; Campbell, 1971; and Thursz, 1970). Concurrently, the greater focus on the problems of *delivery* of medical services has resulted in increasing use of such terms as "health providers" to replace the more traditional terminology of "doctor." Thus, increasingly we speak of the relationship between health *providers* and *consumers* rather than the doctor-patient relationship. Indeed, it is now generally recognized that we are in the early stages of the "age of the consumer." On a variety of fronts the voice of the consumer is making itself heard in a powerful way: for example, Ralph Nader is a symbol of the consumer movement; the executive branch of government has the President's Committee on Consumer Interests; the American Federation of Homemakers is prominent in various consumer legal actions; the National Welfare Rights Organization as a consumer group aims to be the spokesman for the welfare poor; in Philadelphia and in San Mateo, prisoners have brought suit over failure to provide either any or adequate medical or rehabilitative care; and in the health field the consumer movement received particular impetus through the OEO-sponsored Neighborhood Health Centers. (See Sparer et al., 1970.) Indeed, the trend toward citizen control of Neighborhood Health Centers is well advanced and sometimes encouraged by officialdom. This trend toward greater consumer involvement in health affairs is prevalent in a variety of contexts. For example, the following declaration was made at a national conference on rehabilitation:

> The consumer must be a vital and fundamental part of the rehabilitation system — or the system is irrelevant to the recipients of its services . . . consumer participation and the decentralization of programs needs more power to the consumer (National Citizens Conference, 1970).

The experiences of Neighborhood Health Centers may be illustrated by the comments of Martin Cherkasky in reference to the South Bronx Neighborhood Medical Care Demonstration:

> The providers of medical care no longer have the sole prerogative for decision-making and this is all to the good. Health planners cannot understand groups . . . different from their own other than by engaging in the most intimate collaborative planning and management of these joint health care enterprises (Cherkasky, 1969).

A recent statement issued by a group of faculty in Schools of Public Health takes note of the trend by calling for the overall mission of Schools of Public Health to include:

> . . . the facilitation of the development of innovative ways of organizing and delivering community health services on the basis of continuous consultation with both the producers and the consumers of those services . . . the kinds of community health problems which are emerging and becoming dominant are less amenable to technological solutions and more and more require consumer cooperation and collaboration.

The mere use of the term "consumers" to replace "clients" initiates a different perspective. From the perspective of labeling theory of deviance, we can expect differential behavior on a part of perceivers and perceived depending on the labeling used. As a client, on the one hand, the individual delivers himself into the hands of the professional — who presumably is the sole decision-maker regarding the nature of the services to be delivered. On the other hand, when the individual is viewed as a consumer, he is a purchaser of services and tends to be guided by *caveat emptor*. Thus, the switching of labels tends to change the fabric of the social relationships between practitioners in the health delivery system and their clients. The process of social change evidenced by the evolution in relationships from client-practitioner to consumer-provider may be indicative of structural changes in this social relationship. The social construction of the relationships becomes redefined by virtue of the realities imposed in the bargaining and negotiating between client-practitioner versus consumer-provider.

In patient-practitioner relationships power is lodged in the physician and negotiations and bargainings typically do not occur on an equal basis. What we are suggesting is not unlike Freidson's discussion of the patient as "a ward of the system versus the patient as a well-paying customer in a buyer's market" (Freidson, 1970a). In the former, the patient does not have bargaining power to enter into negotiations; in the latter case, the patient may dominate negotiations.

Thus, in consumer-provider relationships, *caveat emptor* implies that the consumer has considerably more bargaining power than formerly. He may, under certain circumstances of a changing social structure of the health system, be able to shop in the marketplace of health care. With the structural relationships undergoing a process of alteration, the behavior of both the professionals and their clientele will be altered. (For a pertinent discussion, see Titmuss, 1963.)

From another conceptual perspective, consumerism tends to take on some of the characteristics of a social movement. "A social movement is a spontaneous large group constituted in support of a set of purposes or beliefs that are 'shared' by the members" (Milgram and Toch, 1969). This definition is somewhat different from Turner and Killian's: "A social movement is a collectivity acting with some continuity to promote a change or resist a change in the society or group of which it is a part" (Turner and Killian, 1972:246). As Toch (1965) points out, a social movement "represents an effort by a large number of people to solve collectively a problem that they feel they have in common." According to this view, the success of social movements depends on the size, organization, and quality of leadership and more upon the extent to which the movement successfully expresses the feelings, resentments, worries, and concerns of large numbers of people and the "degree to which these movements can be viewed as vehicles for the solution of wide-spread problems." Thus, consumerism in health care may be viewed in terms of *shared perspectives*, i.e., as noted earlier, people in similar situations tend to view their problems alike and to evaluate them similarly. It is in this sense that consumerism may take on some of the aspects of a social movement. Thus, as in other movements, there is a redefined perspective; specifically, the role of the client vis-à-vis the professional medical practitioner is altered.

Public statements by health officials and leaders of consumer organizations provide further evidence for viewing consumerism from a social movement perspective. The most outstanding example of this phenomenon is probably the experience of the Office of Economic Opportunity's program of maximum feasible participation by citizens in consumer action programs, particularly in the Neighborhood Health Center's established by OEO. From participation there has emerged a distinct trend toward *control* of such action programs. Thus, consumer involvement and consumer control run counter to the modern thrust of professionalism (Thursz, 1970).

Finally, consumerism manifests itself most prominently in terms of the expression of satisfaction and dissatisfaction with that system in its varying forms. In the usual practice of medicine, patient satisfaction is particularly difficult to express in a way designed to produce change in the system (Notkin and Notkin, 1970). With the system undergoing structural change, however, there may be greater opportunities for producing change through such expressions. The increasing number of published papers concerned with client satisfaction or dissatisfaction with health care is an indicator of the growth of interest in this type of research (Gerst et al., 1969; Henley and Davis, 1967: Kane, 1969). The importance of such studies is not in the intrinsic data presented but rather in their sounding a prelude to something far more fundamental — citizen participation in health care. Accumulation of knowledge concerning consumer satisfaction/dissatisfactions in health and other service-oriented settings will contribute to our understanding of consumerism as a force for changing the professional-client relationships, particularly under bureaucratic settings, and help us understand the social movement aspects of consumerism.

Discussion

This paper is primarily concerned with the issue of changing professional-client relationships consequent to the development of consumerism in our society, particularly in the health field. As the locus of professional-client interaction increasingly takes place in bureaucratic or organizational settings, the nature of the role relationship will be altered. The professional-client relationship tends to be altered as the professional takes into account the client-consumers' wishes, needs, complaints, satisfactions, and dissatisfactions. Eventually, there will be demands for consumer representation on the governing councils of organizations within which the professional and client interact. Just as there is pressure for consumer representation and control at the neighborhood level in the school system, so we can expect that in the medical care field the pressures will continue to build toward consumer representation on hospital boards, prepaid medical care plans, etc.

In addition to consumer representation on governing boards of agencies and institutions delivering professional services, another development may be the employment of an ombudsman. Increasingly, there is greater recognition given to such an office in service-related organizations such as universities, government, and similar enterprises. It is reasonable to expect that the consumer movement will accelerate the adoption of the ombudsman format to mediate differences between professionals and client-consumers.

Viewed from another perspective, it is reasonable to assume that "the legitimate role definers" may no longer be lodged in the particular roles traditionally associated with this function, i.e., professionals. The client, outside of the formal structure of the organization, may become an important factor in such legitimation. As the rules regarding interaction within the organizational or bureaucratic context change, the right to rule on what are the legitimate patterns my shift toward the consumer and away from the professional. Thus, the role-set in the interactive system of an organizational setting, as it relates to professional-client relations and possibly to the organizational division of labor, will tend to change.

Of course, it must be recognized that these changing relationships between the professional practitioner and the client-consumer may vary according to such features as: type of practice, type of physician, type of illness (chronic vs. acute), etc. These variables have always conditioned the nature of the relationship between the doctor and the patient. Furthermore, there are at least two varieties of consumer participation that should be explicitly distinguished:

(1) in the area of health planning and the organization of health services, and,

(2) in the regimen of health care itself, e.g., getting medical checkups, smoking cessation, and other preventive health behaviors that require the client's energies and participation for self-help.

In the former, the processes of change in the professional-client relationship are well-advanced and will undoubtedly continue and perhaps accelerate. In the latter, there may be certain more-or-less enduring features of the traditional model doctor-patient relationship which will set limits on how closely it may approach the pattern of consumer-provided relations in other spheres of consumption — thus limiting the second variety of consumer participation. For example, the client may be in the role of a supplicant; the complex social and psychological process of becoming a client conditions the relationship (Landy, 1965).

As the groups representing "consumers" and the groups representing the health professions confront one another, the interactional processes provide a locus for further study. Attention needs to be given to the forms, content, and symbols used in this interactional process. Out of such observations we can gain better understanding of the underlying processes involved in the changing professional-client relationship.

Although the focus of this paper has been on health, clearly the issues are germane to other areas such as education, employment, housing, etc. Obviously, research is needed on the issues, forces, and processes of consumer involvement in matters typically thought to be the province of the professional and his allies. Perhaps the time has come to modify the standard literature with respect to professionalism and its relationship to clients, or rather consumers. This paper has made an effort to call attention to some of the processes and issues involved in consumerism as these influence and are influenced by social structural changes and the implications for changing roles and relationships of clients and professionals. Clearly, there remain a host of issues to be examined concerning scope, depth, timing, etc., of consumer roles in health decisions.

BIBLIOGRAPHY

Alpert, Joel J., et al.
   1970   "Attitudes and satisfactions of low-income families receiving comprehensive pediatric care." American Journal of Public Health 60 (March): 499-506.

Anderson, R.
   1968   A Behavioral Model of Families' Use of Health Services. Series No. 25. Chicago: Center for Health Administration Studies Research.

Bashshur, Rashid, Charles Metzer and A.B. Worden.
   1967   "Consumer satisfaction with group practice, the CHA case." American Journal of Public Health 57 (November): 1991-1999.

Bloom, Samuel.
   1963   The Doctor and His Patient. New York: Russell Sage Foundation.

Bucher, Rue, and Joan Stelling.
   1969   "Characteristics of professional organizations." Journal of Health and Social Behavior 10 (March): 3-15.

Campbell, John.
   1971   "Working relationships between providers and consumers in a neighborhood health center." American Journal of Public Health 60 (January): 97-103.

Caplan, Eleanor, and Marvin B. Sussman.
   1966   "Rank order of important variables for patient and staff satisfaction with out-patient service." Journal of Health and Human Behavior 7 (Summer): 133-137.

Cherkasky, M.
   1969   "Medical manpower needs in deprived areas." Journal of Medical Education 44 (February): 126-131.

Freidson, Eliot.
   1961   Patient's Views of Medical Practice. New York: Russell Sage Foundation.

1970a Profession of Medicine. New York: Dodd, Mead.
1970b Professional Dominance: The Social Structure of Medical Care. New York: Atherton.
1970c "Dominant professions, bureaucracies and client services," in Rosengren, W. R. and M. Lefton (eds.), Organizations and Clients. Columbus: Charles Merrill.

Gerst, Arthur, Lorraine Rogson and Robert Hetherington.
1969 "Patterns of satisfaction with health plan coverage; a conceptual approach." Inquiry 6 (September): 39-43.

Haug, Marie, and M.B. Sussman.
1969 "Professional autonomy and the revolt of the client." Social Problems 17 (Fall): 153-160.

Henley, Barbara, and Milton Davis.
1967 "Satisfaction and dissatisfaction: A study of the chronically-ill aged patient." Journal of Health and Social Behavior 8 (March): 65-75.

Hochbaum, G.M.
1969 "Consumer participation in health planning: Toward conceptual clarification." American Journal of Public Health 59 (September): 1698-1705.

Inkeles, Alex.
1960 "Industrial man: The relation of status to experience, perception and value." American Journal of Sociology LXVI (July): 1-31.

Kane, Robert L.
1969 "Determination of health care priorities and expectations among rural consumers." Health Services Research 4 (Summer): 142-151.

Landy, D.
1965 "Problems of the person seeking help in our society." Pp. 559-574 in Zald, M. (ed.), Social Welfare Institutions: A Sociological Reader, New York: John Wiley.

Levin, Lowell S.
1969 "Building toward the future: Implications for health education. American Journal of Public Health 59 (November): 1983-1992.

Mechanic, David.
1968 Medical Sociology, A Selective View. Chapters 10 and 11. New York: The Free Press.

Milgram, Stanley, and Hans Toch.
1969 "Collective behavior: Crowds and social movement." Pp. 580-608 in Gardner, Lindsey and Eliot Aronson (eds.), Handbook of Social Psychology. Vol. 4, 2nd edition. Reading: Addison-Wesley.

National Citizens Conference.
1970 People Power: Rehabilitation of the Disabled and Disadvantaged (June), Social and Rehabilitation Services System of Documents. Washington, D.C.: U.S. Government Printing Office.

Notkin, J., and M.S. Notkin.
1970 "Community participation in health services." Medical Care Review 27 (December): 537-543.

Scott, W. Richard, and Edmund Volkart.
1966 Medical Care. New York: John Wiley.

Sparer, Gerald, G.B. Dines and D. Smith.
1970 "Consumer participation in OEO assisted neighborhood centers." American Journal of Public Health 60 (June): 1091-1102.

Thursz, Daniel.
1970 Consumer Involvement in Rehabilitation Social and Rehabilitation Service. SRS-114, System of Documents, Washington, D.C.: U.S. Government Printing Office.

Titmuss, R.H.
1963 "Ethics and economics of medical care." Medical Care 1 (January-March): 16-22.

Toch, H.
1965 The Social Psychology of Social Movements. New York: Bobbs-Merrill.

Turner, R.H., and L.M. Killian.
1972 Collective Behavior. Second Edition. Englewood Cliffs: Prentice-Hall.

Wilson, Robert N.
1963 "Patient practitioner relationships." Chapter 11 in Freeman, H.E., S. Levine and L.G. Reeder (eds.), Handbook of Medical Sociology. Englewood Cliffs: Prentice-Hall.

Wilson, R., and S. Bloom.
1972 "Patient-Practitioner Relationships." Pp. 315-339 in Freeman, H., et al. (eds.), Handbook of Medical Sociology 2nd Edition. Englewood Cliffs: Prentice-Hall.

Beyond a Pious Gesture

Introduction

Previous sections have provided a philosophical framework by which to view the humanization process in health care, a delineation of some of the forces which disrupt the scientific-humanistic health equilibrium, and, an understanding of the psycho-social concomitants of the illness experience. The articles in this section suggest a wide array of vital and compelling strategies towards the enhancement and promotion of humanistic practice. The inherent complexity of the humanistic process in health care makes it unlikely that simple and universally applied cures or panaceas are likely to be found. However, philosophical, causal and analytical understandings of the problems, and positive attitudes and intentions, desirable as both are, come to little if not pursued.

Ultimately, the question that must be answered by practitioners, academicians and society, collaborating in this fertile but yet uncultivated area, is this: is it possible and do we wish — from an educational, programmatic and individual point of view — to develop pragmatic and appropriate strategies and alternatives through which our objective of humane care may be realized? The articles in this section indicate that the answer is yes. Specifically, this entails the careful cultivation and implementation of alternative approaches, methods and programmes to enhance the care of the patient.

We cannot rely solely on the inherent humaneness of the individual practitioners, or the professions to which they belong. Generating humanism is the task of practitioners and educators who can best serve the patient by developing and furnishing organized programmes and standards, and individuals who measure up to them. Without this clearly explicated base for our thinking, we will only be generating "pious gestures."

The first article "The Care of the Patient: Art or Science" by George L. Engel contends that "the care of the patient is as much a matter for science as is the study of disease and that both involve art as well." In this penetrating essay, Engel illustrates the application of the scientific method to the human side of health and illness.

A cogent description of the old and emerging patterns of the doctor-patient relationship is presented in the second article "Compassion in Medicine: Toward New Definitions and New Institutions" by Bernard Barber. The article addresses the question "how shall the move be made more easily toward the newer pattern of doctor-patient relation and the compassion that results from a sense of mutuality?"

The special care programmes needed but too often neglected for the dying patients in our health institutions, are examined by Theodore J. Freedman and Allison J. Stuart in "Caring for the Terminally Ill: One Hospital's Self-Assessment and Solutions."

The importance of using consumer evaluations of the quality of medical care are reviewed by Jay L. Lebow, in our fourth selection "Consumer Assessments of the Quality of Medical Care." Important methodological issues in studies using this approach are discussed and future paths for research are presented. The focus of Lebow's review is the patient's perception of care. He concludes "that once a standard technique is developed, comparisons could be made across types of care, facilities, and physicians to gain insight into what the patient regards as important in care and how he feels about the care he receives."

The need to educate the humanist physician — and other health practitioners — in contemporary society is discussed in the concluding article, in this section, by Edmund D. Pellegrino. In his article "Educating the Humanist Physician: An Ancient Ideal Reconsidered," Pellegrino "intentionally disassembled the ideal of the humanist-physician. This disassembly enables us to understand the full spectrum of meanings within the ideal and to denote educational goals specifically designed to explicate each of the integral components of humanism."

The Care of the Patient: Art or Science?*

George L. Engel

"Affection and zeal may do much, but they cannot take the place of knowledge." Thus spoke John Shaw Billings at the opening of The Johns Hopkins Hospital in 1889 (1). He was referring to the training of nurses. For centuries medicine has stubbornly clung to the view that the study of disease is a science while the care of the patient is an art. And as art is believed to be more dependent on personal qualities than on principles that can be examined and communicated, it is widely accepted that the art of medicine cannot be taught (2). At best it can be demonstrated by precept and example. This dichotomous view that restricts science to disease while relegating the care of the patient to the mystic realm of art is the basis for the frequently voiced complaint that physicians have become too scientific and not sufficiently concerned with patients as human beings. Such complaints have been heard for more than a hundred and fifty years, though from time to time a few have questioned whether the reverse is not the case, whether medicine's neglect of a scientific approach to its human side does not in fact mean that medicine has not yet become scientific enough (3—5).

In this lecture I shall address the question of what in the formal education of the physician is properly classifiable as science and what is classifiable as art. I shall put forth the thesis that the care of the patient is as much a matter for science as is the study of disease and that both involve art as well. In so doing I am taking a lead from Samuel Novey, whose critique of psychoanalysis as a scientific approach to man's inner life and feelings led him to examine what art and science have in common (6). This question is also raised by the noted art historian Gombrich.

For why should we perpetuate that false opposition between science and art which gives to art what is murky, instinctive and by definition inaccessible to rational discussion? It finds no warrant in either psychology or history. Many scientists have testified to the role which creative dreams have played in their work, dreams that were hammered into rational theories by hard and inspired work; many artists, on the other hand use the power of intellect with a lucidity and concentration that rivals that of the scientific pioneer. (7)

From "The Care of the Patient: Art or Science?", by George L. Engel *The Johns Hopkins Medical Journal*, Vol. 140, No. 5, May 1977, pp. 222-232. Copyright © 1977 by the Johns Hopkins University Press. By permission of the author and publisher.
* Presented as the fourth Samuel Novey Lecture in Psychological Medicine, The Johns Hopkins University School of Medicine, November 16, 1976.

Novey emphasizes that while the goal of art is primarily one of aesthetics, of feeling, and that of science one of matters of fact, this does not mean that the arts are to be divorced from the factual or that science may not concern itself with feelings. Attention to a scientific approach to feelings has special pertinence for clinical medicine, the practice of which so much depends on the ability of the physician to understand and to help thinking, feeling human beings. But scientific attention to such matters runs counter to the traditions of physicalist Western science, which has not been inclined to regard feelings, thinking, relating and other distinctively human qualities as proper subjects for scientific study. Novey notes that while the state of mind that seeks specificity of knowledge and of causal relationships is imperative for the physical scientist, such an approach may be more obscuring than revealing when extended into areas where the nature of the problems are quite different, as man's inner experience, his feelings, his spiritual life, and his personal history and development. The last is especially crucial to our thesis, for in medicine the basic strategy for the study and care of a patient is historical. Eliciting and reconstructing the history of the person and of the illness provide the basis upon which much of subsequent clinical reasoning, clinical judgment and clinical decision-making are predicated (8). But because neither the techniques nor the data yielded are readily quantifiable, the clinical approach is deemed more art than science. Such exclusive emphasis on quantification, characteristic of dualistic-reductionistic Western scientific medicine, has been especially important in influencing what is categorized as science and what is categorized as art. Novey writes:

> In these times, when development of "exact sciences" has been stupendous, the very preoccupation with establishing quantifiable principles has become so intense that the broader scope of man's knowledge and interests has tended to become submerged. While the expressed sentiment of the scientist is that he is interested in the quantifiable and is by no means belittling the large areas that may not as yet or perhaps never will lend themselves to quantitative techniques, his actual impact has been different. A kind of arrogance tends to creep in which says that if a body of knowledge is not demonstrated by quantifiable techniques it is worth nothing. More than a little of the frequently observed barriers between the scientist and the humanist derives from this conflict. The psychoanalyst, as well as the medical clinician is often in the position of employing techniques which do not lend themselves readily, if at all, to experimental validation. Very frequently, however, the problems which lend themselves to quantifiable study demand such a reduction of variables and a degree of focusing on areas that can be quantified that the knowledge derived is valueless to the clinician who must meet immediate and pressing problems in his patients (6).

It is precisely this attitude, this arrogance, as Novey put it, that underlies the claim that the care of the patient is primarily an art. For as it involves human transactions that are neither readily quantifiable nor reducible to physicochemical laws, convention assumes that it is therefore not subject to scientific study. And as such it is widely accepted that instruction can be based only on example and adherence to established rules of conduct. In contrast, disease is approached as a matter of science, based on verifiable facts, generalizations and principles, all capable of being communicated to and mastered by the student.

The problem facing medical education is thus one of overcoming conventional attitudes and acknowledging the fact — for it is a fact — that human behavior, feelings, transactions and relationships — and hence patient care — are indeed amenable to scientific inquiry; that it is possible to make precise observations and to provide accurate verbal descriptions thereof, to characterize and classify data, to establish reliability, to draw inferences and to develop hypotheses that can be put to test. As applied to patient care, the initial approach typically is observational and historical, the investigator taking note both of what the patient reports and how he behaves as he recounts his history and as he relates to the physician-investigator. The aim is to establish generalizations that have predictive value and that can provide reliable guides for how the physician should behave under particular circumstances. Once derived, such principles should be capable of being communicated, tested, refined and applied by others.

Before illustrating the application of the scientific method to patient care it is first necessary to specify what that field includes. In the treatment of disease the time-honored precept has been, "Assist Nature and do no needless harm." For patient care a corresponding precept might be, "Assist Human Nature and provoke no needless upset." The doctor's task is to identify the patient's psychological strengths and social resources and help him make best use of them, while at the same time providing the emotional and practical support needed to help compensate for existing weaknesses and deficits. The decisions made and the actions taken must minimize as much as possible needless emotional upset or social disruption.

Patient care encompasses all of the transactions between the patient and the various health providers; it is not the responsibility of the physician alone, though this discussion will be limited to the role of the physician. In practical terms decisions concerning the care of the patient are being made continually by the physician in the course of every transaction with a patient. Their implementation is accomplished through the doctor's behavior, by what is said or done — or not said or done, for that matter, and how. The ultimate goal of a scientific approach to patient care is to render rational and accessible to conscious awareness and reporting the basis for the decisions and the means of their implementation. They should not be personally idiosyncratic, mysteriously intuitive or professionally ritualized, so often the manners in which decisions are made. They must be predicated on reliable data correctly interpreted and on principles amenable to scientific study and validation. Such standards must apply as much to minute-to-minute microdecisions as to more major decisions, whether to linger a moment longer at the bedside as well as when and how to propose open heart surgery.

To illustrate how Human Nature may be hindered, not assisted, and the patient unnecessarily upset, let us turn to an actual incident. From this we may consider how outcome may have been different had the doctor based his decision and behavior on a scientific understanding of human nature.

Case 1

A middle-aged woman with a history of intermittent drinking and fatty liver had been abstemious for several years. She had been feeling relatively well until six weeks before admission when anorexia, fatiguability, weakness, and loss of pep and interest abruptly developed. Her physician concurred with her concern that perhaps her liver trouble had flared up and admitted her to the hospital for liver studies, including biopsy. All the laboratory findings proved unremarkable, and the doctor was now coming to report the results of the biopsy. As we walked to the bedside together he gave me a thumbnail sketch of the case, adding, "I am sure she will be glad to know the outcome of the liver biopsy." He greeted her with a cheerful smile and a wave of his hand, saying, "Good news, Mrs. Jones, the biopsy shows only a *little* fat in the liver. So you can leave the hospital in the morning. I'm sure you'll be glad to get home to your family." The patient smiled faintly but said nothing as the doctor began to palpate her abdomen efficiently while asking, "And how *are* you today?" After momentary hesitation she responded rather wanly, "Pretty good, I guess," but at the same time frowned slightly and raised and then let fall her right hand in the gesture of helplessness (9,10). "Good," said the doctor, "I'm glad to hear that," and walked out of the room with a smile. The patient looked so disconsolate that I lingered behind, commenting, "You don't seem so happy about this." She burst into tears. Encouraged by my interest she readily reported that the anorexia, fatiguability, weakness and decrease in energy had begun abruptly when she learned that her husband of twenty-five years was leaving her for another woman. To me she acknowledged feeling let down, rejected and hurt, but denied that she had resumed drinking. She had hoped to be able to share this information with her doctor, but, she claimed, he gave her no opportunity. When I subsequently inquired, he expressed surprise at the information and amazement at how readily she had revealed it to me.

COMMENT

I shall limit discussion to the decisions bearing on patient care made by the doctor during the few minutes at the bedside. As must be clear, they were predicated on both faulty information and poor observation. Indeed, they were more reflective of the physician's own needs and of a ritualized pattern of behavior than they were responsive to the patient's situation at the moment. The basic requirements of a scientific approach were ignored, presumably because the physician's education had not led him to appreciate that such was possible. We can be confident that his intentions were of the best, to make the patient feel better, and that he would no more knowingly upset his patient needlessly than he would administer a drug contraindicated in liver disease. He was a clinician whose standards would not permit him to make decisions about the treatment of the liver disease without first establishing the pertinent facts. Yet he made decisions about her life without first investigating her current life situation and emotional status. Further, he persisted in his decision in the face of a clear sign from the patient, the hesitant response and the helplessness gesture, indicating that he had overlooked something. Such behavior is equivalent to persisting in the administration of a drug contraindicated in liver disease in the face of jaundice and a palpable liver.

But what, you may ask, does this have to do with science? Is this not merely an example of a physician singlularly lacking in sensitivity, judgment and common sense? (He was in fact a distinguished clinical teacher and investigator, greatly admired by his peers and his students.) The question may perhaps be answered best by reviewing how the scientific method was utilized to establish the meaning of the sign that the doctor had overlooked, namely, the gesture interpreted as indicating a feeling of helplessness. By so doing, I hope to document that clinically relevant psychological phenomena are indeed amenable to scientific study.

First, to describe the gesture more fully, it is typically biphasic. When the gesture is fully developed, both hands are raised fairly briskly to the level of the face, the elbows flexed, the palms facing each other rotated slightly outward, the fingers spread, and the thumb and fingers slightly flexed as though preparing to grasp. This position is held for a second or less, and then the hands fall limply with gravity. Abortive and incomplete gestures may also be seen. Thus the hands may be raised through only part of the arc or only one hand may be lifted a few inches, rotated outward with fingers spread and then allowed to fall back. Sometimes the upward movement of the hands is accompanied by an upward glance, a slight elevation of the brow and lid, and a slight tilt backward of the head. As the hands fall, the face may sag and the body slump as well (9,10).

Certainly this gesture must be familiar to all of you, but whether you consciously equate it with a feeling of helplessness, or even understand helplessness as an affect, is another matter. This is because nonverbal expressions of affects, as gestures, postures, facial expressions and tones of voice, more often evoke feelings than stimulate a conscious intellectual response. Hence, although we may differ in how sensitive we may be to the emotional expressions of others, by and large most of us "feel" before we "know" what the other person is experiencing and communicating. Further, we typically respond to and act on such feelings, at least initially, much more in terms of our own emotional needs of the moment than in terms of the other person's situation. Thus, a nonverbal expression that is threatening, as anger, or demanding, as helplessness or anxiety, may be overreacted to or even screened out altogether lest our own equanimity be threatened. But as physicians committed to helping others in distress, we must go beyond our own feelings to understand what the patient is feeling and trying to communicate. We can do this by developing a scientific typology of gestures, postures and facial expressions and by establishing their relationship to the inner experiences being felt and expressed. Armed with such knowledge, we can deal with them more objectively as signs as well as empathically as feelings. How has this development been accomplished with respect to the feeling of helplessness?

Schmale first formulated the concept of helplessness as an affect in the course of his studies of psychological giving up (11). Put into words, helplessness means, "I give up, there is nothing further I can do, no way I can cope by myself; only someone else or altered circumstances can help." Developmentally Schmale relates the feeling of helplessness to that period from birth to two or three years when the child is totally or largely dependent on adults for even its most elementary needs (12).

The proof of the association of the gesture and the feeling derives from the following sources: (a) verbal expression of helplessness and giving up often is accompanied by the gesture; (b) a familiar metaphor to express the inability to do anything further upon impasse is "to throw up one's hands"; (c) volunteers directed under hypnosis to display through bodily expression the feeling of helplessness characteristically exhibited the gesture. They did not do so in response to the suggestion of thirteen other affects (9); (d) to be held in the arms for the small child means comfort, security and protection. When in distress children characteristically communicate their need for help by looking up and raising the hands, that is, by signalling a wish to be picked up and held. This corresponds to the first phase of the helplessness gesture. Thus, to look up and to raise the hands are behaviors learned early in life to signal a need for help; (e) when active efforts to adjust to a changing environment prove to no avail, life may be preserved by withdrawal, inactivity and disengagement, a biological regulatory process we have termed *conservation-withdrawal* (13,14). We suggest that the muscular hypotonia characterizing this process in primates accounts for the falling of the arms with gravity that marks the second phase of the helplessness gesture.

Thus the helplessness gesture begins with the bodily communication of a wish to be picked up only to be superseded by the hypotonia of conservation-withdrawal as the very reaching for help emphasizes its futility at the moment. In the process the need for help is communicated. The gesture is embedded in both the development biology of the infant-adult relationship and the biological regulatory processes of conservation-withdrawal. As far as we have been able to learn it is a universal gesture.

Let us now return to the clinical example that stimulated this discussion. I leave it to you to decide whether the elucidation of the meaning of the gesture qualifies as science. If you agree, then you must also agree that the doctor's failure to recognize and respond appropriately to the gesture was no more consistent with scientific medicine than would have been his failure to detect and respond appropriately to an enlarged liver. In this instance the helplessness gesture not only indicated the unreliability of the patient's verbal response, "Pretty good, I guess," but it also provided the physician with a second opportunity to consider an alternative diagnosis, namely a depressive reaction. In light of this woman's propensity to resort to alcohol under such circumstances, his failure to interpret and respond to his patient's behavior correctly in fact placed her already damaged liver at greater risk. Clearly here, to have assisted Human Nature would also have assisted Nature.

Let us consider another example. The experienced scientific clinician, familiar with basic pathophysiological principles and how such processes are manifested in clinical terms, is often remarkably successful in drawing correct inferences from a relatively limited set of observations. He is successful because experience has documented for him a high probability that certain clinical phenomena will relate to each other and in turn correlate with particular pathophysiological processes. For example, when a clinician sees a patient propped up with pillows and gasping for breath he immediately thinks of congestive heart failure. This represents a hypothesis, the correctness of which can be quickly tested by further history and examination. Indeed, only a few minutes may be required to establish reliably what for a beginning student might take hours and for a layman be an impossible task altogether. Yet the ability to draw such high-level inferences from relatively limited data and to know how to put them to test is indispensable for the successful identification and correct treatment of disease. The student accomplishes this by painstakingly studying each patient in exhaustive detail in order to establish and understand the correlations that exist between clinical manifestations, laboratory findings and underlying pathological processes. How well that was done at Hopkins in my student days; how poorly it is done in most schools today (15)! Through such exercises, reaffirmed by repeated experience, the scientific physician becomes able at a glance to recognize cardinal clinical manifestations, to derive from them plausible hypotheses and to devise appropriate means to put such hypotheses to test. As a scientist he is meticulous about the reliability and relevance of the methods he uses, diligent in verifying the validity of the data and attentive to alternative hypotheses before he decides upon a course of action. Such commitment to the scientific method is by no means incompatible with the fact that clinical circumstances sometimes require the physician to make decisions and to take action before all the facts are known or all the relevant hypotheses have been formulated and tested. Conscientious adherence to the scientific method is what differentiates the competent physician from the hack and the quack.

These are principles well recognized and observed in the diagnosis and treatment of disease. Do they apply equally for the understanding and care of the patient? They do indeed, and it is only the widely held assumption that such matters are not amenable to a scientific approach that has prevented their inclusion in the education of medical students. Let me illustrate with an example how bits of behavior may also justify drawing inferences pertinent to the care of the patient and how in turn the validity of such inferences can be tested.

Case 2

While serving as visiting professor of medicine at another institution I was asked to interview at grand rounds a man who nine days earlier had suffered a cardiac arrest and had been successfully resuscitated. The only information made available to me was that he was a retired 64-year-old businessman whose arrest had occurred in the parking lot of the hospital. The amphitheatre was crowded and there was barely enough space for the two of us when our patient, a somewhat portly, grey-haired, well-groomed man was wheeled in. In quick succession three bits of behavior were exhibited by the patient. First, in a rapid but nonetheless deliberate manner he carefully scanned the auditorium, his expression changing from a slightly quizzical frown to a faint smile in the few seconds this took. Then apparently he noticed that there was not room enough for both his wheelchair and my chair. As the house officer was attempting to maneuver the wheelchair into place and before I had even sized up what the difficulty was, the patient from his wheelchair began to move my chair. He ended up directing me and the resident until the two chairs were located to his satisfaction. As the interview began I was holding a hand microphone, which after my initial question, I reached over toward him for his response. Then came the third bit of behavior. He at once took the microphone from my hand and responded, gazing alternately from me to the audience. Thereafter it was he, not I, who controlled the microphone. When he had finished saying what he had to say, and only then, he directed the microphone toward me for my next question.

COMMENT

What inferences, if any, may one draw from such a small sample? As with the example of the orthopneic patient referred to earlier, the answer depends on one's fund of knowledge, grasp of basic principles and ability to make reliable observations, this time, however, in the realm of human behavior rather than pathophysiology. Few, I suspect, would disagree that this patient's behavior constituted an effort on his part to establish and maintain control in a new situation. But such a formulation is a mere tautology, comparable to stating that our orthopneic patient was trying to get more air into his lungs. In my own mind I went much further. His behavior, it seemed to me, was all the more remarkable considering the fact that it was displayed a mere nine days after a cardiac arrest. Subdued, passive behavior might seem more plausible under such circumstances. For me, however, his behavior during that first minute immediately brought to mind the behavioral and personality characteristics that many investigators, beginning with Osler in 1896, have reported among patients who develop coronary artery and cerebrovascular disease (16—23). Such a generalization on my part on the basis of merely one minute of behavior is no different than would be my thinking of congestive heart failure and its pathogenesis upon observing a propped-up patient gasping for breath. In both examples, the generalization also predetermines the questions to be asked and the strategies to be invoked to test its validity for the patient in question. In this case we first needed to establish whether this behavior constituted a specific reaction to the situation (that of being presented at rounds) or whether it reflected a more enduring personality style. Further inquiry supported the latter. As he described his hospital experience, the circumstances of his illness, his business career, his personal relationships and family life, his satisfactions and frustrations, and his life style, item after item emerged consistent with such a formulation. His personal account of himself and his life, comprising various episodes, experiences, anecdotes, relationships, expressions of opinion, judgments and self-characterizations, added up to the picture of an aggressive, ambitious, competitive man, always active, busy and planning, preoccupied with deadlines, high standards of performance and self-set goals; a man driven by an inner sense of pressure and urgency; a man who basically felt he could depend only on himself to get the job done and to assure gratification of his own needs. Friedman and Rosenman have popularized this pattern as Type A (20,21). To a remarkable degree his behavior upon entering the amphitheatre accurately reflected many of these characteristics.

On the basis of our developing knowledge of psychological settings that seem especially conducive to sudden death, we entertained a second hypothesis. This premised that the risk of cardiac arrest in the biologically vulnerable Type A person is enhanced when the patient feels or actually is in danger of losing his sense of control over his environment, the more so if preceded by a longer period of discouragement and depression and accompanied by strong feelings of fear, anger or excitement that culminate in a sense of futility or failure (24,25). In this case what emerged on further inquiry was that the patient's carefully laid plans to devote his retirement to "doing his own thing" had been frustrated by his daughter's divorcing and leaving the care of her three-and four-year-old children to the grandparents. To make matters worse, the older boy had become ill. Rather than playing golf and cultivating his many new hobbies he now felt burdened with these unwanted responsibilities as well as disappointed in his daughter. The cardiac arrest occurred on the way to the doctor's office with the four-year-old when a parking space for which he had been patiently waiting was "stolen" by another motorist. He remembers angrily shaking his fist at the motorist, driving off and then nothing more. In the interview this was described as "the last straw." An acute myocardial infarction five years earlier placed him in the group at higher risk for cardiac arrest.

Perhaps you will concede that this is interesting, maybe even persuasive. But the more skeptical among you may still be wondering how such information contributes to more effective patient care. The answer to that question requires a further step. If we are to assist Human Nature, as we earlier defined the goal of patient care, then we must know what these psychological characteristics, so readily established through proper observational and interview technique, mean for the patient and how the physician's approach to the patient may be adopted to minimize distress and encourage confidence and peace of mind. Scientifically, this requires a different level of conceptualization and a different strategy of investigation. It corresponds to explaining orthopnea rather than merely recognizing orthopnea as a cardinal manifestation of left ventricular failure. For orthopnea this requires elucidating the underlying pathophysiology; for Type A behavior, elucidating the underlying psychodynamics.

Basic knowledge of psychodynamics, like basic knowledge of pathophysiology, is best achieved through long term or in-depth study of a few patients. Psychoanalysis has proven to be an especially powerful tool for such purposes. In-depth study of persons exhibiting Type A behavior, whether or not they also have vascular disease, has uncovered a variety of unconscious determinants, the most critical of which is a deep-seated fear of being passive, helpless or dependent. When the response to this is to exaggerate the opposite by striving always to be active, independent and in control of the environment and the people in it, the behavior pattern that evolves may be typically Type A. In such a development the person also becomes his own most severe critic and exacting taskmaster; he continually sets and strives to fulfill higher and higher goals for himself and for others, thereby repetitively subjecting himself to the risk of failure, a failure for which he characteristically takes personal responsibility. By the same token, the deep fear of helplessness and passivity also makes it difficult for him to rest on his laurels; no matter how successful, he must constantly strive for more success (19).

The various developmental factors, biological, psychological and cultural, that may contribute to such an outcome need not concern us here. Suffice to say that failure to take into account these underlying dynamics may have serious consequences for the patient, as the following example illustrates.

Case 3

A real estate salesman in his mid-50s was brought to the Emergency Department of Strong Memorial Hospital with all the classical manifestations of an acute myocardial infarction, confirmed by electrocardiography. While the team was working over him ventricular fibrillation abruptly supervened. He was promptly and successfully resuscitated, much to the satisfaction of all concerned. How fortunate, everyone commented, that he was in Emergency when the arrest occurred; twenty minutes earlier he surely would have died! But ten days later a medical student elicited a different story. A typical Type A who had suffered his first myocardial infarction six months earlier, he immediately recognized his symptoms as those of a heart attack. Nonetheless, he resolved not to call his doctor until he had completed his scheduled work and put his affairs in order for the next day. This he had almost accomplished when his concerned employer herself called and then drove him to the hospital. By the time he arrived symptoms had largely abated and he once again felt relatively in command. Nonetheless, the cardiology team, alerted by his physician, proceeded to minister to him with what the patient experienced as all the high drama of a TV doctor show. At first he was impressed and no little relieved that all this expertise was being directed to his care, though it seemed a bit extreme for one by now feeling as comfortable as he. When the electrocardiogram confirmed the diagnosis he was neither surprised nor upset, for he had already assumed that such was the case. But he was totally unprepared for the intensification of activity that the confirmation of the diagnosis seemed to provoke, culminating in repeated unsuccessful efforts by the intern to perform an arterial puncture. The painfulness of the procedure, distressing as it was, was of less moment to him than was a growing concern that the doctors were neither as experienced nor as competent as he had assumed.

Let us listen to his own words as recorded on tape by the medical student:

> They were having a tough time getting into the artery . . . that drove me crazy . . . I was getting nervous . . . I felt my temperature rising . . . my face was becoming flushed . . . my chest pain began to come back and was getting worse . . . and my arm was killing me. I didn't want to say anything about it . . . so . . . (Why not?) Well, I don't know, I just . . . don't like to . . . you know, I didn't wanna tell 'em that I didn't think, ah, that I knew, he wasn't doing it right . . . they tried here and they tried there . . . the poor fellow was having such a tough time, he just couldn't get it.

Abandoning their efforts the doctors went out to get help, leaving the patient momentarily alone. At first he felt relieved, but anticipating more of the same, he began to feel outrage and then to blame himself for having allowed himself to get caught in such a predicament. A growing sense of impotence to do anything about his situation culminated in his passing out as ventricular fibrillation supervened.

COMMENT

Psychologically speaking, the setting in which this man's cardiac arrest occurred was not different from that reported for the patient cited earlier. But on this occasion the critical events involved the manner in which medical care was being administered. The very fact that all concerned congratulated themselves — and the patient — on his good fortune in being in the emergency department at the time the arrest occurred documents that a relationship between the arrest and the patient's reaction to the unsuccessful efforts at arterial puncture were not seriously considered. Would this have been the case had the cardiology team appreciated the risk factors inherent in the psychodynamics underlying Type A? Indeed, would not a more knowledgeable staff have been attentive to how the patient was responding to the events in the emergency room and have made a more deliberate effort to deal with his feelings before the risk of precipitating a lethal arrhythmia had reached dangerous proportions? For such a risk is very real, as animal experiments have shown, a literature I urge you to review carefully, especially if you are inclined to dismiss these two case reports as merely anecdotal (26—33).

The answer, of course, to both of these questions must be in the affirmative. For just as an understanding of the pathophysiology of left ventricular failure enables one to appreciate the risks of recumbency, physical exertion, or excessive sodium intake, so too does understanding of the psychodynamics underlying Type A enable one to recognize the risks of placing such a person in a passive, helpless position, subject to the domination and control of others. Further, we can readily derive from the dynamics rational strategies to minimize such risks. These in turn can be subjected to test and refined in their application, as is the case with any therapeutic measure. Let me propose, from such principles, a strategy for the care of the Type A patient with a suspected myocardial infarction.

That Type A can be suspected from the patient's reported and observed behavior during the development of the attack and from his interactions with the doctor has already been illustrated in the two cases cited. Once the doctor is satisfied with the reasonableness of such a personality diagnosis, the challenge for the doctor is how to take the firm command that the seriousness of the situation calls for without at the same time mobilizing the patient's deep-seated fear of being helpless and dominated. Somehow the patient must be convinced of the doctor's competence and ability to provide the help he so desperately yearns for but the need for which he cannot easily acknowledge. This can indeed be a delicate balance, especially when the doctor also is a Type A — as many of us are — who feels threatened by patients who resist submitting to professional control. Asked how they would deal with the conflict of a Type A doctor trying to take care of a Type A patient, a group of medical students came up with the following formula: in one way or another the doctor should communicate to the patient, "All my skills and all my knowledge are at your command." An elegant compromise! For thereby each preserves relative autonomy. And although this may facilitate for the patient the illusion that he commands the doctor, in fact the message communicated is that it is the doctor (and surrogates) who are the sole possessors of the critical knowledge and skills.

In practice, care of the Type A patient requires monitoring, as carefully as one monitors cardiac rhythm, where the patient is in his continuing struggle to maintain autonomy while submitting to the demands of treatment. The very fact of the doctor's interest in the patient's concerns over such issues, however expressed, can itself powerfully contribute to a growing sense of trust on the part of the patient, something not easily achieved by Type A people. At the same time the patient's awareness that the doctor is interested in and wants to understand whatever may be contributing to the patient's concerns enables the patient to be more relaxed in relinquishing some of his own need to maintain control. Accordingly, judicious interventions, such as providing the patient with access to a phone or to a visitor, even in the emergency department, so that unfinished business can be resolved, may both relieve the patient's anxiety as well as assure him that he has not been capriciously stripped of all his command. Helpful too are trade-offs, the concession of allowing lesser activities in place of more taxing ones, especially when done in such a way that the patient is given the feeling of participation in the decision to relinquish one activity in favor of another. The interactions between physician and patient in the course of which information and concerns are shared and decisions agreed upon provide the matrix in which the patient eventually succeeds in identifying with the powerful doctor, acquiring thereby the doctor's strengths and sense of competence, rendering him a surrogate instead of an adversary. The patient who says, "I discussed this with my doctor and we decided . . ." often is thereby expressing such a successful identification.

But enough details. I hope what I have provided affords some sense of how a firm grasp of psychodynamics can be put to practical use, even by one who is not an expert in such matters. I need hardly remind you that we are not required to be experts to apply our knowledge of biochemistry or physiology; we are asked only to have a good working knowledge of basic principles. In contrast, the difficulties for both patient and doctor when such principles are ignored are well illustrated in the recently published book jointly written by a patient and his doctor, entitled *A Coronary Event* (34).

I cannot know whether I have persuaded you that the care of the patient, no less than the treatment of disease, is a matter for science and that excellence in both reflects the art with which the physician applies scientific knowledge. The power of dogma is great. More than a hundred years ago Sir William Gull warned against the dogmatism of a too physicochemically oriented "Science, [which] by throwing the light of particular inquiry full in our eyes blinds us for a time to that which lies beyond." (3) The remarkable accomplishments of biomedical research and technology have had just such an unforeseen side effect. And nowhere is this more apparent than in our most prestigious medical centers, where attention to medicine as a human science still receives little attention and less support. Hopkins is no exception. Yet its founding fathers did not plan it so. Sir William Osler, who in 1896 provided the first definitive description of the personality characteristics of angina pectoris victims, early advocated the need for a psychiatric unit as an integral part of the general hospital (35). And when it finally came to pass with the opening of the Henry Phipps Psychiatric Clinic in 1913, he noted that its "very existence in a general hospital indicates the recognition of psychiatry as part of its legitimate work." (36) At the same time he warned against the consequences of isolating psychiatry from the other disciplines: "Isolation means organic inadequacy — each must work in sympathy and in union with the other and all for the benefit of the community — all toward what Bacon calls the lawful goal of the sciences, that human life be endowed with new discoveries and power."

(36) It was William Welch who pursued and ultimately succeeded in implementing these goals when in 1908 he prevailed upon Mr. Phipps to devote his largesse to the establishment of a psychiatric unit (37). Welch was an ardent supporter of the mental hygiene movement and was eager to help create a sound scientific basis for the care of the mentally sick (38). But even in those early days the conception of what should be included in a scientific approach to the mental and psychological was surprisingly broad. Osler urged psychiatry to attend to the needs of the general practitioner for "enlightenment, instruction and encouragement" in the care of the patient encountered in everyday practice (36). His successor in medicine, Lewellys Baker, in 1905 proposed a Psychopathological Laboratory for the investigation of the emotional aspects of patients on the medical wards (39). Such attitudes must certainly have influenced the qualifications sought after in the selection of a chairman for the new department. Adolf Meyer was a far cry from the alienists of his day. Singularly devoted to countering the dogmatism of Cartesian dualism in scientific medicine, Meyer undertook to inculcate in the medical student the notion of man as an adapting organism in an ever-changing environment and of disease as a failure in adaptation (40). His emphasis on the need to take into account all levels of organization, the physicochemical, the biological, the psychological, and the sociocultural, to see man as more than a sum of his parts, as an integrated organism, may be considered as a forerunner of modern general systems theory. Psychiatrists today who advocate psychiatry's adherence to a narrow reductionist biomedical model fail to appreciate what Adolf Meyer so clearly recognized, that the medical model must be broadened, not psychiatry narrowed. Today's crisis in medicine and psychiatry derives from this neglect of a scientific approach to all the dimensions of illness, a direct consequence of the pervasive dogmatism of Cartesian dualism. Truly, as Peabody put it, medicine has not yet become scientific enough (4).

Billings, Osler, Welch, Barker and Meyer were truly prescient in their advocacy of a scientific approach to the human side of health and illness, with all that implies for the quality of patient care. This is part of Hopkins's "Heritage of Excellence," Turner's felicitous term (41). Turner points to "a certain unifying thread that stretches from the seminal ideas of a hundred years ago to what we have today" and urges that we "hold fast that which is good." (42) But we must be careful lest the blinding glare of the dramatic achievements in biomedicine lead us to forget that the founding fathers also included in that unifying thread scientific attention to the human dimensions of illness. The care of the patient as science is indeed a unique heritage of Johns Hopkins. I look to my alma mater now to revive and bring to fulfillment what was so brilliantly pioneered in its early decades. As one of your illustrious faculty so rightly put it, our great medical centers must be more than superb repair shops for broken bodies (43).

FOOTNOTES

1. Billings JS: The plan and purposes of the Johns Hopkins Hospital. *In* Chesney AM: The Johns Hopkins Hospital and The Johns Hopkins University School of Medicine. Vol. I, 1867-1893. Baltimore: The Johns Hopkins Press, pp. 241—255, 1943

2. Ross RS: A letter from Richard S. Ross. Johns Hopkins Med J 137: 238—240, 1975

3. Gull WW: Clinical observation in relation to medicine in modern times. *In* A Collection of the Published Writings of William Whitney Gull. Memoirs and Addresses. Acland TD, Ed. London: The New Sydenham Society, p. 38, 1896.

4. Peabody FW: The care of the patient. JAMA 88: 877—882, 1927

5. Engel GL: Too little science. The paradox of modern medicine's crisis. The Pharos 39: 127—131, 1976

6. Novey S: Psychoanalysis and science. Johns Hopkins Med J 140(5): 233—239, 1977

7. Gombrich EH: The vogue of abstract art. *In* Meditations on a Hobby Horse and Other Essays on the Theory of Art. London: Phaedon, p. 149, 1963

8. Engel GL: Enduring attributes of medicine relevant to the education of the physician. Ann Intern Med 78: 587—593, 1973

9. Schmale AH, Tinling D, and Eby L: Experimental induction of affects. Proceedings of the Seventh European Conference on Psychosomatic Research, Rome, Sept 11—16, 1967, Acta Med Psychosom: 1—8, 1967

10. Engel GL: Signs of giving up. *In* The Patient, Death and the Family. Troup SB and Greene WA, Eds. New York: Charles Scribner, pp. 45—72, 1974

11. Schmale AH: Relationship of separation and depression to disease. I. A report on a hospitalized medical population. Psychosom Med 20: 259, 1958

12. Schmale AH: Needs, gratifications and the vicissitudes of the self-representation. A developmental concept of psychic object relationships. Psychoanal Study Society 2: 9—41, 1962

13. Engel GL and Reichsman F: Spontaneous and experimentally induced depressions in an infant with a gastric fistula. A contribution to the problem of depression. J Am Psychoanal Assoc 4: 428, 1956

14. Engel GL, Schmale AH: Conservation-withdrawal. A primary regulatory process for organismic homeostasis. *In* Physiology, Emotion and Psychosomatic Illness. Ciba Foundation Symposium 8 (New Series). Porter R and Knight J, Eds. Amsterdam: Elsevier-Excerpta Medica, pp. 57—85, 1972

15. Engel GL: Are medical schools neglecting clinical skills? Editorial. JAMA 236: 861—863, 1976

16. Osler W: Lecture on angina pectoris and allied states. NY Med J 4: 224, 1896

17. Arlow JA: Identification mechanisms in coronary occlusion. Psychosom Med 7: 195—209, 1945

18. Kemple C: Rorschach method and psychosomatic diagnosis: Personality traits of patients with rheumatic disease, hypertensive cardiovascular disease, coronary occlusion and fracture. Psychosom Med 7: 85—89, 1945

19. Wolf SG: Cardiovascular reactions to symbolic stimuli. Circulation 18: 287, 1958
20. Friedman M: Pathogenesis of Coronary Artery Disease. New York: McGraw Hill, pp. 78—104, 1969
21. Rosenman RH et al.: Coronary heart disease in the western collaborative group study. JAMA 233: 872—877, 1975
22. Thomas CB: Precursors of premature disease and death. The predictive potential of habits and family attitudes. Ann Interm Med 85: 653—658, 1976
23. Adler R, MacRitchie K, and Engel GL: Psychologic process and ischemic stroke (occlusive cerebrovascular disease). I. Observations of 32 men with 35 strokes. Psychosom Med 33: 1—29, 1971
24. Engel GL: Sudden and rapid death during psychological stress. Folklore or folk wisdom? Ann Intern Med 74: 771—782, 1971
25. Greene WA, Moss AJ, and Goldstein S: Delay, denial and death in coronary heart disease. In Stress and the Heart. Elliot RL, Ed. Mt. Kisco, New York: Futura, pp. 143—162, 1974
26. Johansson G et al.: Severe stress-cardiopathy in pigs. Am Heart J 87: 451—457, 1974
27. Corbalan R, Verrier R, and Lown B: Psychological stress and ventricular arrhythmias during myocardial infarction in the conscious dog. Am J Cardiol 34: 692—696, 1974
28. Corley KC et al.: Electrocardiographic and cardiac morphological changes associated with environmental stress in squirrel monkeys. Psychosom Med 35: 361—364, 1973
29. Corley KC, Mauck HP, and Schiel FO: Cardiac responses associated with "yoked chair" shock avoidance in squirrel monkeys. Psychophysiology 12: 439—444, 1975
30. Lee KT et al.: Experimental model for study of "sudden death" from ventricular fibrillation or asystole. Am J Cardiol 32: 62—73, 1973
31. Harris AS, Otero H and Bocage AS: The induction of arrhythmias by sympathetic activity before and after occlusion of a coronary artery in the canine heart. J Electrocardiol 4: 34—43, 1971
32. Lapin BA and Cherkovich GM: Environmental changes causing the development of neuroses and corticovisceral pathology in monkeys. In Society, Stress and Disease. Vol. I. Levi L, Ed. New York: Oxford University Press, pp. 226—279, 1971
33. Hofer MA: Cardiac and respiratory function during sudden prolonged immobility in wild rats. Psychosom Med 32: 633—647, 1971
34. Halberstam M and Lesher S: A Coronary Event. Philadelphia: J. B. Lippincott, 1976
35. Chesney AM: The Johns Hopkins Hospital and The Johns Hopkins University School of Medicine. Vol. II. 1893—1905. Baltimore: The Johns Hopkins Press, 1958
36. Osler W: Specialism in the general hospital. Am J Insanity 69: 845—855, 1913
37. Chesney AM: The Johns Hopkins Hospital and The Johns Hopkins University School of Medicine. Vol. III, 1905—1914. Baltimore: The Johns Hopkins Press, 1963
38. Flexner S and Flexner JT: William Henry Welch and The Heroic Age of American Medicine. New York: Viking Press, 1942

39. Harvey AM: Creators of clinical medicine's scientific base: Franklin Paine Mall, Lewellys Franklin Barker, and Rufus Cole. Johns Hopkins Med J 136: 168—177, 1975
40. Meyer A: Psychobiology, A Science of Man. Springfield, Illinois: Charles Thomas, 1957
41. Turner TB: Heritage of Excellence. The Johns Hopkins Medical Institutions, 1914—1947. Baltimore: The Johns Hopkins Press, 1974
42. Turner TB: History of medical education at Johns Hopkins. Johns Hopkins Med J 139: 27—36, 1976
43. Frank JD: The faith that heals. Johns Hopkins Med J 137: 127—131, 1975

Compassion in Medicine: Toward New Definitions and New Institutions*

Bernard Barber

What is the meaning of compassion in medicine? What is its place in the art of medicine? If asked to rank compassion as a value in medical care, most physicians and patients would probably consider it as important as science; yet the subject of compassion has received little attention in the medical literature. Since the quality of medical care is a matter of concern to both doctors and patients, it seems worthwhile to explore compassion, an essential constituent of care.[1-3]

It is interesting and perhaps indicative that *Dorland's Medical Dictionary* does not include a definition of compassion. *Webster's Third Dictionary* contains a general definition ("deep feeling for and understanding of misery or suffering and the concomitant desire to promote its alleviation"), which is not irrelevant to the practice of medicine but lacks specific application to it. For a more specific application, I looked at the prospectus for the forthcoming *Encyclopedia of Bioethics*; compassion is not included there either, although some of the articles may refer to it.

But dictionary definitions and other formulas are too simple to explain compassion, since its meaning varies in different societies, historical periods or social situations. Compassion in medicine is best understood as a component of the complex social relations that exist among doctors, patients and the many other participants in health care; the nature of these relations determines the nature of compassion.

Social Relations in Medical Care

As I look at the social relations involved in medical care, I see two separate patterns that define different modes of compassion: the long establised, taken-for-granted and still predominant pattern; and a newer pattern that is gradually emerging along with other social change. The long established pattern, to which most participants in medical care are deeply committed, has a number of consistent characteristics. The doctor is superordinate, the authority, sometimes a person to be venerated. The patient and others are subordinate, respectful, even deferential. The doctor is active, knowledgeable and secure in the system: the patient and others are passive, ill

Printed by permission from *The New England Journal of Medicine*. Vol. 295, No. 17, pp. 939—943, October 21, 1976. By permission of the author.
Supported by the Population Office of the Ford Foundation, New York, NY 10017.
*Delivered as the Nathan Sidel Lecture on the Art of Medicine.
From the Department of Sociology, Barnard College of Columbia University, New York, NY 10027.

informed, frightened and dependent. The behavior of all participants in this system is interpreted in individualistic, psychologistic, states-of-feeling terms; it is not seen to be affected by their roles.[4] Doctors are judged as good guys or bad guys, and patients as good patients or crocks. Shortcomings and delinquencies on the part of the participants are not thought to result from inadequacies in the social system, in which they try hard to play their defined and expected parts, but from personal emotional or cognitive inadequacy.

This individualistic view of the doctor-patient relation is reflected in statements by the late Henry Beecher, a physician who earned high esteem in the medical community. On medical experimentation with human subjects, a practice he was among the first to deplore, Beecher said that whereas "it is absolutely essential to strive "for the subjects' informed consent, a "more reliable safeguard is provided by the presence of an intelligent, informed, conscientious, compassionate, responsible research-er."[5] On the medical profession, Beecher wrote that "no other profession, probably, presents such a generally high level of unselfishness and compassion."[6] (It should be noted that I am not concerned with the accuracy of these statements but with the suggested concepts of doctors and patients.)

In the traditional pattern of doctor-patient relation, the appropriate form of compassion is paternalistic benevolence. It is the physician — active, decisive, individualistically responsible — who defines and dispenses compassionate care. In the treatment of dying patients, for example, Crane has shown that the compassionate doctor of the older pattern would decide to preserve life at all costs.[2] In the newer pattern, on the other hand, social definitions of death and dying have emerged, and the patient, family and others help the physician redefine compassion. Medical compassion in the newer pattern is expressed by actions based on the dying patient's capacity to engage in meaningful social relations.[2]

In this emerging pattern, patients, relatives and others are not so much subordinates of the authoritative doctor but more nearly partners, even "quasi-colleagues," as Talcott Parsons has said.[7] All participants are obligated to be knowledgeable, independent and active. Mutuality and reduction of inequality are preferred to one-sidedness and inequality. Now that members of many socially subordinate categories — blacks, women, young people and students — are asking for greater equality, for the right to participate in the vital decisions that affect them, it is no wonder that patients and other subordinate participants in health-care relations should do so. It is important to remember that subordinate groups are asking for more participation and equality from other powerful professions as well,[8-10] and that the medical profession has not been singled out.

Evidence of the Old and New Patterns

Although Crane's research provides empirical evidence of the two types of doctor-patient relation in the treatment of dying patients, systematic evidence in other types of treatment is not available. Specific data might help to ease the social change that is now in progress, but another kind of evidence can be used to study it.

The paternalism of the older, established pattern of social relations in medical care is manifest throughout the long history of codes of medical ethics.[11] The Hippocratic Oath requires that physicians refuse to grant certain requests — for example, a patient's request for abortifacients — and specifies the doctor's right to determine which confidences should be kept secret. This paternalism is again reflected in the first great modern code, *Percival's Medical Ethics.* Implicit in this code, in the American Medical Association's first code (1847) and in subsequent codes is the assumption that the physician is solely responsible for interpreting the patient's needs.

A move away from the older pattern and toward greater patient participation is reflected in the Patient's Bill of Rights, published by the American Hospital Association in 1972. Under this code, the physician is no longer the sole authority in managing a patient or in deciding what information to give the patient and family. The Bill of Rights states that decision making should be shared with the patient, and it even acknowledges the patient's higher authority in some situations. These principles are officially applied only to patients in hospitals and may not have had much influence even there, but the Bill of Rights clearly departs from earlier codes, which for two thousand years have stressed the doctor's dominance and paternalistic benevolence.

Edmund Pellegrino has written as follows[12]:

> For centuries, physicians were bound together by a common set of moral principles. . . . Physicians who remained faithful to these codes were presumed always to act in the best interest of the patient and the public. Questions of life and death, the choice of medical interventions, and the duties of the profession were left to the good offices of the physician. . . . Physicians rarely debated about the few principles. . . . Their explicit ramifications in practice were considered matters of the physician's personal belief, but not the patient's.
>
> In less than a decade, this comfortable situation has been drastically, and probably irrevocably altered by forces both internal and external to medicine . . . it is no longer possible for the physician to make moral and value decisions for his patient. . . . Physicians must inevitably prepare for a more open dicussion of moral choices and values with patients and society. They must recognize that medicine's traditional moral authority is no longer universally accepted.

Effects of Inequality in the Doctor-Patient Relation

Most people brought up in an established system of social relations can be expected to adhere to it. They will tend to exaggereate its virtues, to minimize its apparent defects and to oppose changes that may detract in some way from themselves. Many people still maintain that the traditional system of medical care has been entirely satisfactory in providing compassionate concern for the needs of patients, but there is at least one type of doctor-patient interaction, the use of human subjects in medical experiments, in which selfless concern has not always been demonstrated.

In 1970, my colleagues and I interviewed 337 research physicians in two typical biomedical-research institutions, a community teaching hospital and a university hospital and research center.[13] In an effort to estimate the researchers' concern with the rights and welfare of human subjects, we asked them to judge two detailed, hypothetical research protocols.

In the first proposal, designed to reflect concern with the relative risks and benefits to the subjects, we asked the researchers to evaluate a study of the effects of radioactive calcium on bone metabolism in children with a serious bone disease. The proposal stipulated that, if successful, the investigation might eventually benefit the group of subjects with the disease, but it could not possibly benefit the control group of healthy children. In addition, the experiment would slightly increase the likelihood that leukemia would develop in both groups. Fifty-four per cent of the physicians who responded disapproved of the study no matter what probability of an important medical discovery was given; however, 16 per cent approved when the probability of success was given as one chance in 10, and 30 per cent approved various higher probabilities.

The second proposal was designed to reflect concern with the subjects' right to informed, voluntary consent. The protocol described a study of pulmonary function in adults undergoing a routine hernia operation. So that the researcher could obtain the data, the subjects would remain anesthetized for an additional half hour. The chances of postoperative complications such as atelectasis and pneumonia were likely to increase slightly. This proposal, unlike the first one, did not mention informed consent, and 24 per cent of the respondents objected to the study on that basis. Another 40 per cent objected after a probe by the interviewer, but 17 per cent said that informed consent should not be required.

Thus, a substantial proportion of these physicians did not show concern for the welfare and rights of patients. In our view, these defective standards resulted from strong emphasis on the autonomy of the individual physician, from insufficient mutuality with patients and other physicians and from the attitude that the doctor knows best. But morality and compassion have essential social components. The individual physician, who may not know what is best, would be helped by greater participation in a moral community of patients and fellow doctors.

Now that the newer pattern of more equality and mutuality in the doctor-patient relation is emerging, many physicians have expressed the fear that the authority required for effective treatment will be eroded or even destroyed. In many types of interactions, it is difficult to distinguish authoritarianism, in which those in power assume the sole right to make value decisions, from just and necessary authority, in which those in power share the right to make decisions in the area of their expertise.[14] In doctor-patient relations, the authority needed for effective medical treatment is implied by the physician's scientific knowledge, which the patient may not share. But even as one acknowledges an irreducible imbalance in the prerogatives of doctor and patient, one must assert the necessity for continual justification of this imbalance. Doctors must establish, more clearly than many of them do now, that acquired knowledge, rather than personal superiority, underlies their authoritative declarations. Paradoxically, they may have to admit more readily to uncertainties, since greater equality requires greater communication of weaknesses as well as strengths.

It may not be easy to achieve a better communication of the grounds for claiming and receiving authority and trust; for some physicians, trained in and committed to the older pattern of doctor-patient relation, it may be impossible. Similarly, some patients may prefer the older type of interaction. Social change always involves the possibility of considerable personal strain. In medical-care relations, the strain should be eased by the tendency of doctors and patients to select, informally, the old or new type of relation.

I hope it is clear that, when I speak of greater equality as a constituent of the new pattern, I do not mean absolute equality. Most patients are asking only for more participation in the vital decisions that affect them. A few may react against any degree of authority, but occasional over-reaction is found in many areas of social protest. It should not be confused with the basic phenomenon, the wish for less-than-total but still essential change.

Possible Agents of Change

How shall the move be made more easily toward the newer pattern of doctor-patient relation and the compassion that results from a sense of mutuality? I should like to say a bit about four groups that could ease the transition: established medical professionals; young people just entering the profession; the government; and friendly but critical outsiders. Each of these groups has a special part to play, and each has unique problems and responsibilities.

The weight of authority and the consequent power to change medical-care relations lies with the established medical professionals. The same influence that is used to maintain the present system could provide an invaluable resource for changing it. With some important exceptions, however, most medical professionals are in favor of the existing system. Their conservativism is not surprising; it is the established, prestigious participants in any system who maintain its stability and resist forces that press for change. This situation may be intensified in the medical profession, which has a proud and committed establishment. Nor should one expect that simply because the medical profession is innovative, even radical, in terms of scientific change, it would also be open to a social change that would affect its authority and autonomy. Perhaps because of of the scientific nature of the medical profession, which for the past few generations has selected its leaders on the basis of their commitment to the autonomy of scientists, it will be particularly unsympathetic to a social pattern that seems to subvert individualism. It is not surprising that many members of the establishment resent, not only lay participation in medical care, but peer control as well. Belief in the moral rightness of the older, personalistic pattern has apparently produced this resentment.

What of the young people who are just entering the profession? Perhaps they will show more social creativity. Young people are often responsive to new ideas and social patterns, and members of this young generation have probably had a more egalitarian background in their families, schools and peer relations than the older generation had. An aspect of their medical training that suggests some movement toward the newer values in medical-care relations is the availability of courses in medical ethics. In a recent survey, Robert Veatch found that during the past six years, nearly all of 107 American medical schools have introduced courses in or related to ethics.[15] In addition, many schools now offer conferences, workshops, case discussions and lectures on ethics. However, the effectiveness of these efforts is difficult to predict.

Comparable movements, such as the attempt to persuade medical students to spend less time on "hard" subjects and more on psychiatry, comprehensive care, community medicine and preventive medicine, have been much less successful than their proponents hoped. Medical students are bright and ambitious; they have no difficulty ascertaining which subjects are taken seriously by the prestigious, senior members of the faculty. How many take medical ethics seriously? How many are committed to the teaching of ethics in the same way that they are committed to their scientific research? More important, how many key faculty members treat ethical issues in discussions of basic scientific and clinical issues, to which medical ethics are often applicable? Only six of the ninety-seven respondent schools in Veatch's survey teach ethics as a required course. Forty-seven offer elective courses in it, but the percentage of students enrolled in them has not been reported. In the remaining schools, definitive ethics courses are not given. Since medical students tend to concentrate on required scientific and clinical courses, classes in ethics may not lead to greater sympathy for changes in medical-care relations unless senior instructors show concern about ethics in their classes, research, rounds and discussions, and at the bedside.

The third agent that may facilitate social change is the government. Although it has had an increasingly important financial role in the health-care system, the government has had little direct involvement in patterns of medical-care relations. Although indirect effects of its financial involvement are feared, the government has not challenged the accepted authority of the medical profession by requiring more egalitarian relations between clinicians and patients. The call for full patient access to medical records, for example, has come, not from the government, but from members of the medical establishment — important exceptions to the more numerous conservatives I have mentioned.

Regarding the use of human subjects in medical experiments, however, the government has used the power of the purse to increase patient participation. Since 1966, federal funding for medical experiments on human subjects has required local peer review and proper standards of informed consent and risk-benefit ratio. The government at first advised and now requires lay participation on all local peer-review committees. Two years ago, the government established the National Commission for the Protection of Human Subjects of Medical Behavioral Research and stipulated lay membership on the Commission. Although nonprofessionals have by no means predominated on peer-review committees or the National Commission, their advocacy of higher standards and practices in the use of human subjects has had some influence. As another sign of the times, a Symposium on Patients' Rights in May, 1976, was sponsored by the Health Services Administration.

But even direct government intervention in medical-research relations has produced only slow and minor changes; indeed, the government has sometimes simply insisted on standards and procedures that were already proclaimed by the medical profession. It is important to remember that the greatest influence on the National Institutes of Health regulations for medical investigation with human subjects probably came from its own research community.

Although the government has hardly revolutionized social relations in medical care, there has been much resistance to government initiatives, and some have predicted that the new regulations would "kill science," even though medical researches have made great advances during the past thirty years of federal funding. Government participation is not necessarily destructive; with the creative co-operation of the medical profession, government initiatives in the area of social relations could have a constructive effect. There could be some loss of autonomy and individualism, but it would not be the end of the medical world.

The final agents of change that I have mentioned are the "friendly outside critics" — a group of economists, sociologists, philosophers, religionists and journalists who believe that changes in the established pattern of medical-care relations are desirable, and that these relations should permit greater equality and the compassion that is an outgrowth of equality. They also believe that the practice of medicine, like any specialized vocation in contemporary society, is too important to the society to be regulated solely by the specialists.

Some of these critics have failed to base their assertions on a close study of medical-care relations or to take into account the hard complexities, dilemmas and tragedies that are sometimes unavoidable in health care. Yet an increasing amount of good research and moral sensitivity among the friendly critics suggests that their help in smoothing the course of social change may be considerable. Another favorable development is that these outsiders are beginning to be accepted by the medical establishment, even though there is occasional ambivalence or excessive expectation.

Conclusion

My topic has been compassion in medicine. Though I may appear to have gone the long way around the barn, compassion must be seen as an aspect of social systems and relations. These systems and relations are now changing, and so are the valued modes of compassion. Though they cannot be the only agents of this change, I hope that medical professionals will assume a larger and more creative role in it, and that they will achieve as fine a record in interpersonal medicine as they have in scientific medicine.

FOOTNOTES

1. Fox RC: Experiment Perilous: Physicians and patients facing the unknown. Glencoe, Illinois, Free Press, 1959
2. Crane D: The Sanctity of Social Life: Physicians' treatment of critically ill patients. New York, Russell Sage Foundation, 1975
3. Lally JJ, Barber B: "The compassionate physician": frequency and social determinants of physician-investigator concern for human subjects. Social Forces 53:289-296, 1974
4. Henderson LJ: Physician and patient as a social system. N Engl J Med 212:819-823, 1935
5. Beecher HK: Ethics and clinical research. N Engl J Med 274:1354-1360, 1966
6. *Idem*: Experimentation in Man. Springfield, Illinois, Charles C Thomas, 1958, p. 23
7. Parsons T: Research with human subjects and the "profession complex." Daedalus 98:325-360, 1969
8. Freidson E: Professional Dominance: The social structure of medical care. New York, Atherton Press, 1970
9. Rosenthal DE: Lawyer and Client: Who's in charge? New York, Russell Sage Foundation, 1974
10. Barber B: The social control of the professions: toward a solution of an ethical crisis, Columbia University Seminar Reports. New York, Columbia University Press, 1976
11. Berlant JL: Profession and Monopoly: A study of medicine in the United States and Great Britain. Berkeley, University of California Press, 1975
12. Pellegrino ED: Medical ethics, education, and the physician's image. JAMA 235:1043-1044, 1976
13. Barber B, Lally JJ, Makarushka JL, et al: Research on Human Subjects: Problems of social control in medical experimentation. New York, Russell Sage Foundation, 1973
14. Slack WV: Patient power: a patient-oriented value system, Computer Diagnosis and Diagnostic Methods: Proceedings of the Second Conference on the Diagnostic Process held at the University of Michigan, June, 1970, Edited by JA Jacquez. Springfield, Illinois, Charles C Thomas, 1972, pp 3-7
15. Veatch RM, Sollitto S: Medical ethics teaching: report of a national medical school survey. JAMA 235:1030-1033, 1976
16. Friedenwald H: The ethics of the practice of medicine from the Jewish point of view. Johns Hopkins Hosp Rep 318:256-261, 1917

Caring for the Terminally Ill: One Hospital's Self-Assessment and Solutions

Theodore J. Freedman and Allison J. Stuart

Since the work of Dr. Elizabeth Kubler-Ross and Dr. Cicely Saunders, there has been steadily increasing interest in the needs of terminally ill patients by health workers and the general public. In Canada, the work of Dr. Balfour Mount at the Royal Victoria Hospital in Montreal has been recognized and followed with great interest. However, despite the fact that seventy percent of all Canadians die in health-related institutions,[1] hospitals have formalized very few programs to meet this evident need. In fact, in all of Canada, only two palliative care units exist.

Stimulated by the example of the Royal Victoria Hospital,[2] the patient care and utilization committee and the administration of Mount Sinai Hospital, a 573-bed teaching hospital in Toronto, decided to undertake a study to determine if the hospital was meeting the specific needs of terminally ill patients and their families. An ad hoc committee for the total care of the terminally ill was formed in 1975, bringing together representatives from the departments of family and community medicine, medicine, nursing, obstetrics and gynecology, psychology, psychiatry, radiological sciences, rehabilitation medicine, social work, and surgery; the Baycrest Centre for Geriatric Care; the board of directors; the house staff; the hospital chaplain; and a doctoral student in psychology working in the field of death and dying. The committee was chaired by the associate executive director. In order to accommodate such a large, diverse group and make decisions on this difficult subject, the ad hoc committee established three subcommittees — a retrospective study subcommittee, a prospective study subcommittee, and a questionnaire subcommittee — and requested them to collect data on the hospital's established mode of care for terminally ill patients.

The retrospective study subcommittee initially conducted a review of deceased patients' medical records and then interviewed these patients' next of kin. Although the results obtained were not helpful in formulating a data base, the subcommittee did discover significant information that indicated a need for change in the system. For example, it was found that medical staff members were not documenting information dealing with the patients' emotional needs and social interactions, or what was told to the patients and their families and by whom; this deficiency in charting was considered to be a signal of a possible break in communications between

Reprinted, with permission, from *The Hospital Medical Staff*, published by the American Hospital Association, Vol. 7, No. 2, February 1978, pp. 7-12. By permission of the authors.

the physicians and the nurses. Also, as a result of information obtained from the next-of-kin and from the Montreal[3] program, a bereavement follow-up program was started to help these individuals cope with their loss and grief.

The prospective study subcommittee initially began its study by having three committee members interview the terminally ill patients, their families, and the hospital staff, but the members' other responsibilities did not allow them sufficient time to complete all the interviews required. Thus, they designed a questionnaire to be completed by the staff caring for the terminally ill patients.

This study also indicated the difficulty of accumulating information on the terminally ill. For example, although some very important facts were revealed, the information was obtained from a sample of only twenty persons. Furthermore, the nursing staff was reluctant to identify a patient as being terminally ill. Kubler-Ross also encountered the denial of death among her medical colleagues when she sought dying patients to help: "It suddenly seemed that there were no dying patients in this huge hospital."[4] However, the committee also recognized this problem as partially being due to the difficulty in defining the term "terminally ill," as well as the staff's reluctance to use this term.

The questionnaires highlighted several significant problems: There was a lack of communication between the medical staff and the nursing staff as to what information the patient had been given. A total of 45 percent of the nurses responsible for the patients did not know what the patient knew. This concurred with the lack of information in the medical record, as found by the retrospective subcommittee. When the staff was asked, "Does the patient appear to be in pain?," they replied that forty-five percent of the patients seemed to be in moderate to severe pain. More complete information on the patients' conditions is required before a conclusion can be reached. However, the ad hoc committee was concerned with these findings, and an additional study is necessary because recent literature[5,6] indicates that pain can be managed to a greater degree. As Mount has written, "Before all else, palliative care must mean excellent symptom control, achieved by a health care team skilled in clinical pharmacology."[3]

The ad hoc committee plans to focus its attention on these recent findings and develop appropriate programs.

Concurrent with the activities of the other two subcommittees, the questionnaire subcommittee developed a questionnaire to obtain the views of all categories of staff dealing with terminally ill patients. An excellent response was received. Seventy-five percent of the respondents were medical or nursing staff. Some of the findings were as follows: Eighty percent of the respondents believed that terminally ill patients should usually or always be told their diagnosis and prognosis. This compares with the prospective study in which thirty percent were told they were terminally ill; thirty-five percent were provided only with a diagnosis; ten percent were told an unrelated diagnosis; twenty percent were not applicable due to level of unconsciousness; and five percent were not told anything. More than ninety percent of the respondents stated that they would want to know the details of their prognosis if they were terminally ill, yet only sixty-two percent would definitely want their families to know. This compares with the prospective study in which seventy percent of the families knew the patient was dying; five percent knew the patient was in poor condition; and twenty-five percent were provided with a diagnosis.

Fifty-three percent of the medical staff felt that their preparation for dealing with the emotional needs of the terminally ill patients had been adequate. However, seventy-four percent felt that they could cope with the emotional needs of the dying patients and their families in an adequate way.

They did indicate though that they needed the most help in dealing with the families of terminally ill patients (forty-three percent) and the least in working with other medical (eight percent) and nursing (nine percent) staff members. Twenty percent wanted assistance in coping with their own feelings and seventeen percent wanted to know more about talking to the patient himself.

Only sixteen percent of the medical staff thought that a special geographic unit devoted to the care of the terminally ill should be established in the hospital, and sixty percent thought that a special team should be established to help staff with the total care of the terminally ill patients.

One surprising and disappointing statistic was that only twenty-one responses (thirteen percent) were received from the 160 house staff members, and this occurred after repeated efforts were made by the president of the house staff and the chairman of the ad hoc committee. A similar study done at the Royal Victoria Hospital received a response rate of twenty-five percent from house staff.[7] The low response rate was not expected because it is the house staff who deals most directly with the patient, his or her family, and the rest of the health care team on a day-to-day basis. Further study is required to determine the reasons for the poor response.

As a result of the findings, a consultation team was established to assist all hospital staff in caring for the terminally ill. This team consists of representatives of the departments of medicine, nursing, nutrition and food services, occupational therapy, physiotherapy, psychiatry, and social work, and the hospital chaplain. Initially, the chairman of the ad hoc committee is acting as chairman of this team.

The consultation team has concentrated thus far on the preparation of a protocol for the care of terminally ill patients. It outlines the most common problems encountered and suggests appropriate actions. The protocol is standardized for use by the entire health team for any terminally ill patient, but it can be modified to meet the unique needs of each patient. Its format is similar to the nursing care plans used by the hospital, in order to facilitate its acceptance and use.

The protocol consists of two sections: (1) two pages attached to each medical record of a terminally ill patient, providing the reader with appropriate care alternatives for common problems; and (2) a learning folder located at each nursing station, with two divisions: (a) physical-psychological-neurological, and (b) psychological-social-spiritual. The learning folder contains both articles and specific recommendations for treatment of the common problems of the terminally ill. One section, for example, provides recent articles on the appropriate management of pain in terminally ill patients. The protocol will also be circulated to the house staff members of the hospital.

Proper management of pain is an important consideration. Shephard wrote: "Perhaps because persistent pain is so debilitating and demoralizing . . . the control of pain is frequently the key to good palliative care. Pain can be controlled when an interdisciplinary team attacks the physical, social, psychological, and spiritual components of pain in a milieu that is supportive of that patient."[8] The consultation team will attempt a similar approach.

A number of the committee members and the majority of the medical staff initially believed that an acute care general teaching hospital need not segregate terminally ill patients in order to provide them with a high standard of individualized, concerned care. Thus, the committee is working toward providing these patients with a quality of care that meets their varied and specific needs within the medical/surgical services to which they are admitted. Prior to the reports of the subcommittees, no evidence indicating that this objective was not or could not be met existed. However, the evidence now indicates that the very specialized needs of terminally ill patients could be more fully met within a unit devoted to them. Therefore, the ad hoc committee will soon tackle the issue of establishing a geographic unit for their care.

However, the responsibility extends beyond that of the hospitals. Eventually, it will be necessary to effect changes in the medical schools, for example, because hospitals are the recipients of the students and staff that are products of today's curriculum. It will also be necessary for society to change its attitudes before we can rightfully expect that the needs of the terminally ill will be met.

The ad hoc committee at Mount Sinai Hospital has been successful in implementing several programs to help the medical and hospital staff meet the needs of terminally ill patients and their families. Their goal has been to establish an environment that emphasizes improvement of the quality of life remaining during the patient's stay.

As is evident from the Mount Sinai experience, hospitals and their medical staffs can play a major role in changing the traditional way of dying. A caring hospital can always delve into "quality of patient care" issues and, by so doing, improve the level of total patient care being provided. Although the results of studies are not always what one wishes to find, the process of constant evaluation and reevaluation is vital if the hospital wants to maintain a high standard of service.

FOOTNOTES

1. Statistics Canada. *Vital Statistics Bulletin, Vol. 3.* 1973, p. 61.
2. Aitken, J. Fond farewell — compassion and honesty for the dying. *Weekend Magazine.* June 21, 1975.
3. Mount, B.M. *Report of the Pilot Project (Jan. 1975-Jan. 1977), Palliative Care Service, Royal Victoria Hospital, Montreal.* Montreal: Royal Victoria Hospital, 1976.
4. Kubler-Ross, E. *On Death and Dying.* New York: MacMillan Publishing Co., Inc., 1969.
5. Mount, B.M., and others. Use of Brompton mixture in treating the chronic pain of malignant disease. *Can. Med. Assoc. J.* 115:122, July 17, 1976.
6. Melzack, R., and others. The Brompton mixture: effects on pain in cancer patients. *Can. Med. Assoc. J.* 115:125, July 17, 1976.
7. Mount, B.M., and others. Death and dying attitudes in teaching hospitals. *Urology.* 4:741, Dec. 1974.
8. Shephard, D.A.E. Principles and practice of palliative care. *Can. Med. Assoc. J.* 116:522, Mar. 5, 1977.

Consumer Assessments of the Quality of Medical Care

Jay L. Lebow

This review will focus upon one type of care quality evaluation study: the consumer evaluation of care. First, a brief summary of different methods of study of medical care quality will be presented in order to show some perspective on how complex medical care quality assessment is. Second, studies available dealing with consumer evaluations of care will then be reviewed, followed by a general methodological discussion of the consumer evaluation method. Finally, some areas for future research will be presented.

Research efforts assessing medical care quality have vastly expanded in recent years. While the notion of evaluating the results of care to improve techniques is as old as medical science itself, actual objective study of the care situation by objective evaluators of the care process is a recent development. Few studies of medical care quality predate 1950 and not many articles were written about this topic before 1960. Most studies in the area have been conducted in the last five years.

Of the several possible reasons that more study has recently been made of consumer opinion about care, the most important are the increased concern with patient care among members of the medical profession, the introduction of social scientists with their sophisticated sampling techniques in medical care settings, a growing questioning by the general population of the infallibility or homogeneity of medical care, the increased availability of government money for the study of all aspects of health, greater general concern with objective measurement of all phenomena, the development of large organizations (*e.g.*, insurance plans) interested in carefully monitoring the health and care of their clients, and the increased prominence of health as a factor in the quality of life.

Methods of Medical Care Assessment

Despite the increasing interest in medical care quality, no consistent approach to research has yet to emerge in this area of study. Numerous ways of studying medical care have been proposed and tested. However, it is difficult to compare results of studies since the models underlying the methods employed study care quality from such different perspectives. Furthermore, the existence of such widely diverse institutions as the general hospital, small clinic and private office, each with their own forms

From *Medical Care*, Vol. XII, No. 4, April 1974. By permission of the author and publisher.

This review was initiated as part of a project supported by a grant from DHEW — National Center for Health Services Research and Development, #5-T01-HS 00049 03.

of care, makes the generation of general assessment model difficult. Evaluation is also complicated by the fact that the health care institution, the medical staff, the patient and the patient's family all have different perspectives on the nature of medical care. It is, then, no wonder that review of the field reveals for the most part piecemeal, uncoordinated studies which pay little attention to other work done.

A review of approaches to care quality measurement is beyond the scope of the present article. Approaches to care quality measurement have been reviewed and criticized amply elsewhere.[10-13] In general, reviews have stressed four types of studies of care: structural process, end result, and impact. The structural approach considers only the organization of the care institution in terms of employee time use, client time use, smoothness of functioning, and the like. Since simulation rather than actual data is most commonly used in structural studies, they are probably of little general significance for the study of quality. Most often, the intent of such studies is to determine what structure is best for what situation without invoking any other quality measures.

The process approach[13] to medical care assessment includes more use of data than the structural approach. In process studies, the actual care process is the focus of study. Lee and Jones,[27] in what has become a classic definition of the process criteria, suggested that quality includes simply those medical practices which are recognized and taught by the leaders of the medical profession at a given time in a given population setting. For those who adhere to such a definition, to assess quality is to compare health personnel behaviors with a set of model behaviors. To do so, model behaviors must be specified; often this is a most difficult task. Model behaviors, also, vary in definition across place and time. Thus, the relativity of good medical care is a central problem for assessment. Good care today may be poor care tomorrow. For these reasons, the itemization of elements of "good" care for process evaluation has been largely stymied. Only recently has a group at Yale University in a series of studies attempted to establish such a list of specific physician responses to specific difficulties to serve as testable criteria for care quality studies.[16,33,34]

Either staff records or observer records are the source of data and the records often are scored according to previously determined criteria of "good" care. Use of observers[7, 32] allows for more direct assessment of the care-giving situation, complete data, and the opportunity to consider interpersonal as well as physical aspects of the situation. High potential reactivity and cost are its drawbacks. On the other hand, staff records[8, 15, 30] are more prone to be inaccurate, incomplete, and biased, do not usually include any interpersonal contact information, and may not always be available. However, they are cheaper and less likely to be reactive since the practitioner evaluated does not necessarily know his performance is being measured as he almost always must when observed. In choosing a data source using the process approach, the cost, the availability, and the quality of records should be considered.

End-result measures[26], [29], [31], [37] focus on the result of care rather than the process of care. Donabedian[11] referred to this method as the ultimate validator of other quality measures since care quality, in the final analysis, is what is done for the patient. The assumption is made that given similar cases, better care should result in a shorter illness period, reduced death rate, reduced pain, and changes in other personal health aspects of the patient. The advantages of the end-result method are its objectivity and immediate concern with patient welfare. Its major difficulties are the problems of longitudinal follow-up, *i.e.*, lost subjects, expense, and the possible action of unknown interfering variables that might be confounded with the quality of the care given.

Impact,[10] a fourth approach, concentrates on the effect of care on the overall community setting. The major advantage of such an approach is that it includes individuals who have not seen physicians in the overall quality judgment thus providing more generalizable results. The incidence of individuals needing care who do not receive care at all is an important factor in assessing quality of care. Preventive care also is stressed in impact evaluations. Difficulty in reaching individuals, in indexing health of a community, and in comparing different populations constitute the major problems in the impact approach.

The multiplicity of notions of what "quality care" implies has led to numerous and divergent approaches to measuring care quality. Because of the differences in definitions and theoretical models, each approach delimits its own notion of quality, excluding certain other aspects. Consequently, each approach has major strengths and weaknesses in attempting to tap overall quality. No one approach can be said to include the totality of aspects of medical care. Approaches must be used together to give a profile of the quality of care in an institution. Many different dimensions of care need to be assessed in an evaluation of overall quality and quality can only be assessed as an entity by the use of a multitrait multimethod matrix[4] with careful delineation of each individual aspect of quality.

Patient Evaluations of Medical Care

A fifth approach to the evaluation of medical care and the focus of this review, is patient perception of care. Although such measures are often grouped with process or end-result of care (*e.g.*, Donabedian[11]), such labeling is an oversimplification since an individual's perception of care is more complex that either process or end-result evaluation. Experience in previous medical care situations, the mood of the questioned individual during the care situation, the time of assessment and other factors affect the patient's perceptions but are not accounted for in process or end-result assessment. Patient perception of care differs somewhat from the "objective" aspects of care, and can be considered separately.

Measures of consumer perception of quality have not been employed in many studies. This may be due to fears of possible inaccuracies of patient opinion by researchers, to the low status of patient opinion among physicians,[23] or to the newness of quality of medical care research. However, some studies have used patient opinions. Kisch and Reeder[23] in a study of welfare patients' attitudes, utilized a simple patient interview to discern whether patients felt they had received the care they sought. Only seventy-five per cent of the patients responded affirmatively, indicating that not all patients received care they sought.

Fisher[17] utilized medical students to conduct 30-minute interviews with chronically ill patients in another clinic study. In addition to demographic characteristics, Fisher asked such things as: whether or not patients experienced pain before coming to the clinic (60% — yes), whether or not they experienced improvement (55% — yes), whether or not they were aware of their prognosis (60% — yes), their feelings about the physical facilities, and their average stay (4-1/2 hours). In addition, patients rated physicians' characteristics and rank-ordered what they desired in a medical care center. The most desirable qualities sought in a center were, first, good doctors, followed by well-trained staff, information from doctors, personal interest in patient, pleasant staff, and privacy, in order of importance. Satisfaction was found to be related to improvement in condition, personal interest of the staff in the patient, and explanation received about their conditions. Also, patients who rated the clinic negatively on one item tended to do so on other items as well.

In another clinic at Meharry Medical College, Birch and Wolfe[3] employed a patient-satisfaction questionnaire and a series of projective devices to measure attitudes of patients. Through the direct questionnaire method, high satisfaction with care was found (exact satisfaction rates were not reported). The authors felt that there was less patient satisfaction indicated by the projective technique although no actual scoring of projective material was done.

Other studies have focused on patient evaluation of hospital care. Cartwright[6] and Duff and Hollingshead[14] employed some satisfaction measures in studies of hospital care. Both studies focused on sociological interaction, however, and measured patient satisfaction only secondarily. Cartwright's study done in England found higher rates of satisfaction with physicians than Duff and Hollingshead's study conducted in America.

Houston and Pasanen[20] employed a patient satisfaction questionnaire with patients recently discharged after at least a two-day stay at a large hospital. Thirty-one per cent were hospitalized for a check-up, the others for some illness. Care was evaluated extremely favorably, with the highest ratings given to physician and nurse care. Most dissatisfaction involved the patients' feeling that, although the physicians did understand their physical problems, they did not adequately disclose the nature of the illness to the patient. The overall level of patient satisfaction with care was found to be related to the amount of information received by the patient. Overall,

83 per cent felt improved from the hospitalization and no patient felt worsened by it, although 17 per cent did feel they would be reluctant to return to this hospital again if they had to.

Abdellah and Levine[1] utilized a checklist to measure patient satisfaction exclusively with hospital nursing care. Satisfaction levels were found to be directly related to the amount of care given.

Two studies have focused on patient evaluation of group practice. Freidson[18] in a questionnaire study of group practice in a hospital, found that patients rated technical accuracy, personal interest of staff, and accessibility as the most important factors in care. Although most patients indicated that all three factors were present at the hospital studied, suggesting satisfaction, 46 per cent of patients still used some outside facility for obtaining additional care. Thus, the group practice, while rated highly, was not exclusively used by patients, possibly indicating some deficiency and again indicating the need for multiple measures of care quality.

Weinerman[39] found that only 7 per cent of the patients evaluating two medical group practices were dissatisfied with care. Personal interest of the physician, accessibility of the service, and convenience for the patient were rated as important factors in judging care.

In one of the few outpatient care quality assessment studies, Jolly et al.[22] found in a study of outpatient care of pregnant women that although very few visits were rated "not nice," a large percentage (40%) of the patients complained that the explanations offered were poor. No overall satisfaction measures were employed in this study.

Finally, in a more general frame, Hulka et al.[21] created a Thurstone-type patient-satisfaction scale featuring subscales of professional competence, personal qualities of staff, and cost/convenience of treatment. However, there have been no results of the use of this device reported.

Parent Evaluations of Pediatric Practices

Four studies have employed opinion survey techniques to study pediatric care, with parents of the patient serving as prime source of information about care. DeCastro and Amin[9] studied satisfaction in an ambulatory pediatric unit headed by two pediatricians, newly reorganized within a hospital serving lower class patients. By both direct questioning and a sliding scale assessment, satisfaction was rated very high.

Korsch, Gozzi, and Francis[24] in a study notable for rigor of technique, evaluated tapes of the patients' visits, reviewed medical charts, and conducted two interviews with parents of children visiting an outpatient emergency clinic. One interview was performed immediately after care was received, the other after a substantial time had passed. A novel attempt in care evaluation studies was made when they tried to measure the extent of crossinfluence between measures by employing different combinations of the measuring devices with different subjects. Three groups were used.

One group received all the techniques except tape recording, one group all but the postvisit (first) interview, and one all the techniques. The semistructured interviews were aimed at gathering information about the S's perception of the doctor-patient interaction, the S's satisfaction, and the S's compliance with the doctor's directions. Eight hundred follow-up (second) interviews and 293 postvisit (first) interviews were conducted. Seventeen physicians were the source of care under study.

Results of the study showed no cross-influence of the use of one technique of evaluation on other measures. Satisfaction levels by Ss were high or moderate (76%) whether or not tape recording or first interview were used. The order in which the measures were taken did not appear to affect the results. Other results showed that social class, education, doctor seen, length of visit, and diagnosis did not have any relationship to satisfaction with the visit. Patients expected that physicians would be friendly and communicative and when the physicians did not meet their expectations, satisfaction was decreased. Failure to confirm an expectation to learn the cause of a disorder, to receive an X-ray, injection, cure, medication, or hospitalization all substantially reduced satisfaction levels.

Despite the importance of the patient's expectations, only 35 per cent of expectations and 24 per cent of main worries were, in fact, mentioned to the physician in the visit. The least well-educated Ss were less likely to discuss these matters. Also mothers often reported blaming themselves for their child's illness, predicted their child's disease category well, and restricted the child's activity from the disorder beyond the physician's instructions. Satisfaction and reported compliance were also not found to be related. In an analysis of the visit tapes, the physicians were found to be in control of the interaction and often did not listen to the mothers. Also, the mothers asked few questions although many of the mothers reported that they wanted to ask more questions of the physician. Thus, from these results, a need for altered interactions with mothers seems to be indicated. The methodological precision and vast scope of the Korsch, *et al.* study might well be emulated by other researchers in the area.

Lerner, Haley, Hall, and McVarish[28] employed a parent-satisfaction questionnaire in conjunction with other measures to assess quality of care in an experimental pediatric ward. In the experiment, parents aid in giving nursing care to their children. As assessed through an interview technique, parents were found to be quite satisfied with the innovative care measures. Given the high level of consumer satisfaction with care in other studies, a further evaluation of satisfaction with the innovative care procedures as compared to a control group receiving more typical care seems necessary.

In a study comparing the quality of medical care received by children in a hospital with the care received by children at home, Shah *et al.*[36] also used parent opinion as a major source of data. Preferences for a type of care were found to be related to the type of care received; those who received care which was novel desired it more. The use of consumer satisfaction evaluation here and in the Lerner et al.[28] study as a means to assess the desirability of innovative procedures are good examples of how such measures might most constructively be employed. Assessments of care quality probably can be best employed in studies designed to compare different care-giving approaches rather than in those constructed solely to give an overall numerical quality of care index for one type of care or institution.

Methodological Issues

Several methodological issues must be raised in a consideration of the medical care quality assessment studies using the patient's perspective. Research in the area will not be of the highest quality until some of these issues are discussed, understood, and acknowledged, if not corrected. Reliability of data is one basic issue in patient-satisfaction studies. Reliability refers to whether the results would be identical if the research were redone. The only report so far on the reliability of patient opinion is in the Korsch et al.[24] study, which indicated little difference between judgments of parents about their child's care at different times. Unfortunately, other studies have not collected data in a manner in which reliability could be assessed.

The degree of concurrent validity between different assessment methods of patient satisfaction is a second methodological issue in patient-satisfaction studies. In a test of concurrent validity, the degree of agreement between different measures of the same entity (here satisfaction) is assessed. Although this question could be studied by multimethod tests,[4] such analyses rarely have been made. Most studies have used only one single assessment device. Birch and Wolfe,[3] however, did test for concurrent validity. They used a projective evaluation of care by getting patient reactions to Thematic Apperception Test-like cards depicting medical-care-giving situations. The authors found that the projective test indications of satisfaction with care were lower than the direct questioning indications. However, since projective methods are subject to serious methodological questions themselves,[35] they do not offer a good methodological contrast for direct questioning in a test of concurrent validity. However, the hint offered by Birch and Wolfe's projective data should not be ignored.

The extent to which patients' reports reflect their true feelings about care is another issue. Reactivity, changes in response because the subject knows he is being evaluated, may cause responses to inaccurately reflect patients' real opinions. If the study is internally initiated, the subject may want to please the evaluator; if externally initiated, the subject may want to present his physician in a favorable light. The extent of reactivity is difficult to measure and thus far has been ignored. Exploration of these issues is necessary. One way might be to use unobtrusive measuring devices[38] which would be less subject to reactivity.

Another major methodological concern about perception of care studies is the extent to which patient opinions accurately reflect care given. Here the issue is external validity.[5] It is unfortunately quite difficult to assess whether patient opinion does reflect the quality of the care. The only method indicating the validity of such data is comparison of care perception of the patient with other approaches to care assessment, *i.e.*, structure, process, outcome, and impact measures. Although few actual comparisons have been made, a number of studies show that patient surveys and other more "objective" care measures do not correlate highly. Ehrlich, Morehead, and Trussell[15] found patient evaluation of care to be considerably higher than physician ratings of records of the same care. In an ingenious study, not of satisfaction but concerned with consumer reports, Gordis *et al.*[19] found that parents of pediatric patients claimed they followed physicians' instructions more than they actually did. Patients' urine samples were examined for presence of prescribed drugs over a period of days; compliers were defined as showing 75 per cent or higher positive drug-present rates, noncompliers, 25 per cent or less. A large difference was found between patient verbal statement about drugs taken and the drug content revealed. Of the 22 per cent who were noncompliers, 75 per cent defined themselves as compliers. A similar false reporting of compliance was found in a study of penicillin use in acute streptococcal cases by Bergman and Werner.[2]

Such results should make one cautious about use of patient evaluation, although the findings do not imply that patient opinions should be abandoned as a source of data. Patient questionnaires remain the best method of reaching important aspects of patient care such as how the patient perceived and felt about care. Ratings by others would not be able to assess certain aspects of the interaction between medical personnel and the patient.

One explanation for the difference between patient opinions and other measures that was found in Ehrlich, Morehead, and Trussell's[15] study is that physician raters may have been more rigid on criteria of care or may have utilized different criteria for assessing care than patients. In the Ehrlich, Morehead, and Trussell[15] study, patients were not necessarily "wrong" in their perceptions. That patient opinion was higher, however, does indicate strongly the need for both patient opinion and other evaluations of the care situation to provide a complete view of care given.

The Gordis[19] and Bergman and Werner[2] studies indicate that in a reactive situation where the attending physician inquires about the extent to which directions were followed, inaccurate information is likely to be obtained. Gordis[19] however, utilized an unusual sample (rheumatic fever patients on constant medication who are expected to occasionally fail to follow directions) which may have increased the rate of distortion. The implication is not that possible inaccuracies in data should be ignored; distorted responses may be present, especially in relation to questions in which some responses are more socially desirable than others, such as the following of physician recommendations. In general, information gathered from patients should be checked against other sources whenever possible. When assessments employing differing devices agree about the quality of care, the confidence in the validity of each of the individual measures increases. Unfortunately, even such measures are not infallible checks on validity. Different aspects of care may be different in quality and have differential import across evaluators. Without an absolute measure of quality as a comparison, a perfect, one-step, validational check on all data is unavailable.

Another issue in patient-satisfaction surveys involves the variability found in the data. In most recent studies, especially those conducted in settings in which most care is actually given (*i.e.*, nonclinic setting) consumers have consistently rated care very highly. While such a finding is interesting in itself, indicating a high satisfaction of the population with their physicians, the lack of variability might be due to the way in which questions are worded. Given the numerous instances of this finding under different conditions, however, this seems unlikely. Lebow[25] found similar high approval of care quality by parents of pediatric patients who were given two different sets of extremes for responses on an eight-point scale. The study also found this similarity in response across quite different aspects of the care situation. In general, it seems likely that the high approval of care is not an artifact of the specific questioning procedure.

The lack of variability in patient evaluation also makes the validity, *i.e.*, if such measures reflect real patient feelings, of such measurement questionable. Do most patients really approve of their physicians? Do they give an accurate picture of the way care is given? The question does remain as well how useful is a measure that shows no variance. If everyone is equally approving of care, one can only get reassurance from such findings and not much indication about what to do aside from continuing one's present procedures. More exploration of why this variance is so low and whether it might be raised in certain situations is needed. The possibility does exist that the high approval rate may be simply the product of most patient's ability to choose their own physician, thus finding one of whom they will approve. Many consumers, such as those in small communities and rural areas, however, may not have such a choice. Studies comparing patient satisfaction in groups with free access to many physicians versus those severely limited in choice should prove interesting. Also why such drastic lowering in approval rate in some studies is found[14] needs to be explored. The difference may be due to a difference in quality of care, or populations under study, or measurement techniques. Clear exploration of these factors in care evaluation needs to be made.

The most basic methodological difficulty in the area of medical care assessment by patients is that researchers cannot do true experiments in such settings. In true experiments,[5] one is able to randomize subjects into different groups, give precise treatments to different populations, and compare the results. Given the nature of most medical care, such treatment is impossible. Almost all patients selectively choose their physicians and the instance in which the patient is randomly assigned to a physician clearly is atypical of medical care. Thus, the researcher is left with the choice of studying atypical care or forgoing the ability to randomly assign patients to groups. In the first case, the study merely reflects something about impersonal clinic care and not the type of care the average American receives. In the second, it is possible that different populations exist in the experimental groups before treatment is given, thus invalidating the results.

Suggestions for Further Research

Above all in consumer assessment of care quality, more standardization of method by different researchers seems to be needed. When each researcher uses his own scale, it becomes difficult, if not impossible, to compare results across studies. Once a standard technique is developed, comparisons could be made across types of care, facilities, and physicians to gain insight into what the patient regards as important in care and how he feels about the care he receives.

Much of the research is needed because of method problems in present studies. Reliability of patient evaluation needs to be assessed. Also the concurrent validity of different methods of measuring patient satisfaction and of patient satisfaction with other methods of measuring care effectiveness need to be pursued in all types of situations. Interviews, questionnaires, and other methods assessing patient opinions need to be compared. The use of unobtrusive measures of care satisfaction[38] might be useful. For example, some unobtrusive measures might be: measuring the rate of return to a physician, obtaining patient opinion without informing the patient that his satisfaction level is being evaluated, or having the patient discuss care with a stooge of the experimenter — who would rate the patient's satisfaction.

Multimethod multitrait designs are suggested for all investigations. In multimethod evaluation, one might use questionnaires, checklist items, open-ended items, interview and projective devices, and comparative ratings of care by the same individuals. More than one assessment should be made at a time in more than one way to determine whether the judgment is typical. It might be interesting to ask, for example, whether the satisfaction with physicians is any higher than satisfaction with one's plumber or market, or how such matters are related. Such questions might show whether it was just a matter of the self-selection involved in choosing one's physician that causes such high assessments of care. Comparing consumers' satisfaction in areas with large choice of physician versus those in which there is little choice might further answer this question. Comparisons of all satisfaction measures with process, end-result, and impact assessments also are needed. In all such multitrait multimethod comparisons, it is, of course, important that each aspect of quality of care itself be carefully delineated.

Studies of the care quality evaluation by the patient should also be done in which one attempts to randomize the sample of patients across groups as much as possible. A comparison of the same physicians treating randomly assigned patients and patients who were intentionally coming to them might further illuminate the question of the effect of patient selection. Other attempts might look at satisfaction in instances rated by other physicians as poorer care situations.

Attempts might also be made to isolate doctor, nurse, and institution characteristics and to see how they affect the perception of care. Projects comparing patient satisfaction under different methods of care (HMO versus group versus solo care, or prepaid versus fee-for-service) also need to be conducted. It is also important in further pediatric research to compare parents' and child's evaluation of care and specifically to assess the accuracy of parental judgment of quality. Above all, however, there is a need for more studies of the general issues and more coordination of the studies that are done. The greatest present needs are for careful studies comparing methodological approaches to larger samples of patients, staff, and institutions than have thus far been employed. The area of patient evaluation of satisfaction with care and the whole area of care quality assessment is vitally important and will continue to increase in importance in the near future. It is thus important that good methodology for evaluation be applied in consumer assessment measures. Toward this end, more social scientists expert in methodologically sound assessment should be consulted in evaluation efforts.

FOOTNOTES

1. Abdellah, F.G., and Levine, E.: Development of a measure of patient and personnel satisfaction with nursing care. Nurs. Res. 5:100, 1957.
2. Bergman, A., and Werner, R.: Failure of children to receive penicillin by mouth. N. Engl. J Med. 268:1334, 1963.
3. Birch, J., and Wolfe, S.: A pretest of a patient-satisfaction study as a step to ghetto consumer evaluations of health care. Unpublished, 1972.
4. Campbell, D.T., and Fiske, D.W.: Convergent and discriminant validation by the multitrait multimethod matrix. Psychol. Bull. 56:81, 1959.
5. Campbell, D.T., and Stanley, J.: Experimental and Quasi-experimental Designs for Research. Chicago, Rand McNally, 1963.
6. Cartwright, A.: Patients and their Doctors. New York: Atherton Press, 1967.
7. Clute, K. F.: The General Practitioner: A Study of Medical Education and Practice in Ontario and Nova Scotia. University of Toronto Press, 1963.
8. Daily, E.F., and Morehead, M.A.: A method of evaluating and improving the quality of medical care, Am. J. Public Health, 46:848, 1956.
9. DeCastro, F., and Amin, H.: An ambulatory pediatric unit: consumers' satisfaction. Clin. Pediatr. 9:445, 1970.

10. DeGeyndt, W.: Five approaches for assessing the quality of care. Hosp. Adminis. 000:21, Winter, 1970.
11. Donabedian, A.: A Guide to Medical Care Administration: Volume II — Medical Care Appraisal. New York, American Public Health Association, 1968.
12. Donabedian, A.: Evaluation of the quality of medical care. Milbank Mem. Fund Q. 44:166, 1966.
13. Donabedian, A.: Promoting quality through evaluating the process of patient care. Med. Care 6:181, 1968.
14. Duff, R.S., and Hollingshead, A.B.: Sickness and Society. New York, Harper and Row, 1968.
15. Ehrlich, J., Morehead, M.A., and Trussell, R.E.: The Quantity, Quality, and Costs of Medical and Hospital Care Secured by a Sample of Teamster Families in the New York Area. New York, Columbia University School of Public Health and Administrative Medicine, 1961.
16. Falk, I.S., Schonfeld, H.K., Harris, B.R., Landau, S.J., and Milles, S.S.: The development of standards for the audit and planning of medical care, I. Am. J. Public Health 57:1118, 1967.
17. Fisher, E.: Patients' evaluation of outpatient medical care. J. Med. Educ. 46:238, 1971.
18. Freidson, E.: Medical care and the public case of a medical group. Annals of the American Academy of Political and Social Science 346:57, 1963.
19. Gordis, L., Markowitz, M., and Lilienfeld, A.: The inaccuracy of using interviews to estimate patient reliability in taking medicine at home. Med. Care 7:49, 1969.
20. Houston, C., and Pasanen, W.: Patients' perceptions of hospital care. Hospitals 46:70, 1972.
21. Hulka, B., Zyzanski, S., Cassel, J., and Thompson, S.: Scale for the measurement of attitudes toward physicians and primary medical care. Med. Care 8:429, 1970.
22. Jolly, C., Held, B., Caraway, A., and Prystowsky, H.: Research in the delivery of female health care: recipient's reaction. Am. J. Obstet. Gynecol. 110:291, 1971.
23. Kisch, A., and Reeder, L.: Client evaluation and physician performance. J. Health Soc. Behav. 10:51, 1969.
24. Korsch, B., Gozzi, E., and Francis, V.: Gaps in doctor-patient communication, 1. Doctor-patient interaction and patient satisfaction. Pediatrics 42: 855, 1968.
25. Lebow, J.: Evaluation of an outpatient pediatric practice through the use of consumer questionnaires. Unpublished manuscript.
26. Leonard, R.C., Skipper, J., and Wooldridge, P.J.: Small samples field experiments for evaluating patient care. Health Serv. Res. 2:46, 1967.
27. Lee, R.I., and Jones, L.W.: The Fundamentals of Good Medical Care. Chicago: University of Chicago Press, 1933.
28. Lerner, M., Haley, J., Hall, D., and McVarish, D.: Hospital care by parent: an evaluative look. Med. Care 10:430, 1972.
29. Lewis, C.E., Resnik, B.A., Schmidt, G., and Maxman, D.: Activities, events, and outcomes in ambulatory patient care. N. Engl. J. Med. 280: 645, 1969.
30. Morehead, M.A.: The medical audit as an operational tool. Am. J. Public Health 57:1643, 1967.

31. Payne, B.: Continued evolution of a system of medical care appraisal. JAMA 201:536, 1967.
32. Peterson, O., Andrews, L., Spain, R., and Greenberg, B.: An analytical study of general practice in North Carolina. J. Med. Educ. 31: Part 2, 1956.
33. Schonfeld, H.K., Falk, I.S., Lavietes, P., Landwirth, J., and Krassner, L.: The development of standards for the audit and planning of medical care: good pediatric care. Am. J. Public Health 58:2097, 1968.
34. Schonfeld, H.K., Falk, I.S., Lavietes, P.H., Milles, S.S., and Landau, S.J.: The development of standards for the audit and planning of medical care: pathways among primary physicians and specialists for diagnosis and treatment. Med. Care 6:101, 1968.
35. Sechrest, L.: Testing, measuring and assessing people. In Borgatta, E., and Lambert, W. (Eds.), Handbook of Personality Theory and Research. Chicago: Rand McNally, 1968, p. 529.
36. Shah, C.P., Robinson, G., Kinnis, C., and Davenport, H.: Day care surgery for children: a controlled study of medical complications and parental attitudes, Med. Care 10:436, 1972.
37. Shapiro, S., Williams, J.J., Yerby, A., Denson, P.M., and Rosner, H.: Patterns of medical use by the indigent aged under two systems of medical care. Am. J. Public Health 57:784, 1967.
38. Webb, E., Campbell, D.T., Schwartz, K., and Sechrest, L.: Unobtrusive Measures. Chicago: 1966.
39. Weinerman, E.R.: Patients' perceptions of group medical care. Am. J. Public Health 54:880, 1964.

Educating the Humanist Physician:
An Ancient Ideal Reconsidered

Edmund D. Pellegrino

We must understand what man is, for he is the subject matter of the science of medicine for whom it is promulgated. To understand him is to understand the world, for he is similar to the world in his construction. He is the microcosm, the macrocosm in miniature.

—*The Caraka Samhita*[1]

In the growing litany of criticism to which our profession is increasingly exposed, there is one that in many ways is more painful than all the rest. It is the assertion that physicians are no longer humanists and that medicine is no longer a learned profession. Our technical proficiency is extolled, but in its application we are said to be insensitive to human values. We are, in short, presumed to be wanting as educated men and as responsive human beings.

The assertion is painful because there is some truth in it. Moreover, it comes from those who experience our behavior — our students and our patients. And, in truth, our art is indeed in danger of being engulfed by its technological apparatus. But most painful of all, the assertion strikes at the reality that alone gives authenticity to our profession — our unique charge to answer the appeal of a sick and anxious person for help that is both competent and considerate.

The criticism is especially poignant for medical educators, at whose door much of the responsibility is laid. We are told that we neglect the teaching of human values and the *art* of medicine; that in our zeal for science we ignore liberal studies; and, most telling of all, that the patient care we provide in our teaching hospitals and clinics is itself dehumanizing.

Even our friendlier critics are alarmed by the recent trend to shorten medical education. They fear that our haste will further erode the liberal education of future physicians and thus accentuate the dehumanization of the student and the depersonlization of the patient. These anxieties reach crucial dimensions when viewed against the context of the erosion of personal elements inherent in medicine's increasing institutionalization and specialization.

The terms *humanism, compassion,* and *liberal education* are all shibboleths easily employed to advance one's own political, social, or educational ideologies. Without some clear display of the anatomy of these concepts, physicians will only respond with defensive denial, while their critics will yield to enraptured denunciations. As always, the patient will be victimized by an exchange of diatribes, rebuttals, and contumely. Worst of all, we will

From, *The Journal of the American Medical Association*, Vol. 227, No. 11, March 18, 1974, pp. 1288-1294. Copyright 1974, American Medical Association. By permission of the author and publisher.

miss the opportunity to reexamine these terms and redefine them in their contemporary setting.

There is indeed a genuine and urgent dilemma. Society has the right to require that physicians be competent, that they practice with consideration for the integrity of the person, and that some of them also be educated men who can place medicine in its proper relationship to culture and society.

Medicine enjoys a unique position among disciplines — as a humane science whose technology must ever be person-oriented. Its practitioners are, therefore, under an extraordinary mandate to live and work within a humanistic frame. What does it mean to educate a humanist physician in comtemporary society?

To answer this, we must first examine more closely what we mean today by this ancient ideal. The term *humanist* is too often appended to the term *physician* in an intuitive and altogether imprecise fashion. I suggest that the ideal encompasses two essential but distinct sets of components — one affective and one cognitive. These differ markedly in content; the one does not guarantee the other. In the best examples they are complementary, but they may also be in conflict. Each requires a different mode of learning and teaching.

The failure to make these distinctions leads to pretension, on the one hand, or unfilled expectations, on the other. In either case, the concept loses credibility, and this must be prevented in these times when medicine faces unprecedented demands on all its humane components.

The Physician as Humanist — A Bimodal Concept

So much feeling surrounds the idea of the physician as a humanist that it is somewhat precarious to attempt a clarification, for clarification requires a dissection of the major components of the idea of humanism. Thus, we run a risk of generating an antinomy where ideally none should exist. Nonetheless, much confusion will arise if we fail to comprehend fully the differences in the two concepts that are inextricably associated with any discussion of humanism — medical or otherwise.

Two concepts of the idea of humanism were recognized by Aulus Gellius, the second-century grammarian, when he spoke of the meaning of the word *humanitas,* from which "humanism" was later derived. He distinguished *humanitas* — education and training in the "good" arts — from a "good" feeling toward all men. *Humanitas* is more properly subsumed under the Greek term *paideia* — an educational and cognitive ideal; and the "good" feeling — what we would call compassion — is more akin to the Greek concept of *philanthropia.*[2]

Following Aulus Gellius, we can discern the same two ideals when embodied in the term *humanism in medicine.* One, the cognitive, deals with the physician as a man, a cultural being possessing ideas, values, and modes of expression in word and art. The other, the affective, concerns the feeling of the physician for the person-as-patient experiencing the existential trials of illness. Together, these ideals enable the physician to understand his science and also to identify with the humanity of those he serves.

These two ideals must further be built on a firm basis of technical competence. Without clinical craftsmanship, the physician-humanist is without authenticity. Incompetence is inhumane because it betrays the trust the patient places in the physician's capacity to help and not to harm. Throughout this essay, I shall assume that education in clinical competence always proceeds, *pari passu*, with the affective and cognitive elements of humanism, our major concern.

The "Compleat Physician" is one who is capable in all three dimensions: he is a competent practitioner; he is compassionate; and he is an educated man. To use the classical terminology, he combines *techné* with *philanthropia* and *paideia*. Few men can perform with perfection, or even adequately, at all three levels. We must repress the tendency to apotheosize our profession by expecting all physicians to excel in all three. No educational formula, ancient or modern, can make of everyone who studies medicine the renaissance men or polymaths some vainly hope for.[3] A more realistic educational goal is to open the possibility for all students and practitioners to live in some measure at each of these three levels. Competence and compassion are clearly requisites for each physician if he is to meet his social responsibilities adequately. The extent to which he must also be an educated man is more variable and less intimately related to his social utility.

The Affective Components

Compassion: Its Meaning and Erosion. — Of the two components of humanism, the affective is more frequently mentioned by today's critics of medicine. They decry the lack of compassion they perceive in the care of patients. Compassion is most often equated with humaneness and even with humanism. What do we mean by compassion as an affective attribute of the humanist physician?

Com-passion means co-suffering, the capacity and the willingness of the physician somehow to share in the pain and anguish of those who seek help from him. It connotes some understanding of what sickness means to another person, together with a readiness to help and to see the situation as the patient does. Compassion demands that the physician be so disposed that his every action and word will be rooted in respect for the person he is serving. Compassion is reflected in a disposition to "feel" along with the patient. When it is genuine, compassion is unmistakably sensed by the patient and it cannot be feigned. It is not to be confused with pity, condescension, or paternalism. Clearly, compassion is an affective and behavioral characteristic that bears little relationship to a cognitive appreciation of any of the humanities. Nor is it altogether synonymous with the political or activist bias of many students and young physicians, however well-motivated they may be, to help the socially and economically disenfranchised members of our society.

Potent influences in modern medicine and society now conspire to erode and even extinguish compassion. Among the most influential are our fascination with technology, gadgets, and instruments; the inherent depersonalizing influences of our highly institutionalized social structures;

the replacement of care by individuals with care by the "team"; the thrust of a scientific medical education that focuses on man-the-object-of-study; and, finally, a medical education that itself is fraught with rigidities and does little to help the student develop his own humanity.

Can the affective components of humanism — the *philanthropia* of Gellius — be assured in the education of physicians? Formal education would appear to be of limited value, since humaneness and compassion are not disciplines to be learned in classrooms. Indeed, whenever we study man, even his affective and behavioral components, we must in some sense make him an object and distort him. This is true even of those disciplines, like the social sciences and the humanities, that look at the conscious and imaginative dimensions of man's existence. They may help us to understand humanity abstractly, but not to behave compassionately. We must remember with Jung that "the patient is there to be treated and not to verify a theory."[4]

Compassion In the Student-Teacher Relationship. — Before the student can begin to feel the plight of his patient as that of a person seeking help, he must develop a fuller insight into his own developing humanity. The affective education of the student starts with the means most significant for him — the humanization of his medical experience. By dealing in a personalized and compassionate way with the special circumstances into which a medical education places young people, the teacher may forestall that subtle erosion of sensitivities that is a genuine danger of too much immersion in the study of man as an object of science.

The student-teacher relationship has many similarities to the patient-physician relationship. In both circumstances, one person is seeking help from another who is presumably wiser and has power over the petitioner. Both student and patient must face personal challenges in emotionally trying situations. When the teacher helps the student in a compassionate and understanding way, he illustrates how the student can in turn give the same understanding to the patient, who is dependent on his humaneness as the student is dependent on the teacher's.

The rigidity of current curricula and testing methods, as well as the trial-by-ordeal proclivities of some faculty members, are perceived by many students as "dehumanizing." This experience erodes their own capacities for humane relationships with patients. Granting a certain inevitable hyperbole in such assertions, the only effective way to inculcate compassion is to practice it. In each of their contacts with students, patients, and even with experimental animals, the faculty must exhibit genuine care. The clinician-teacher has truly awesome responsibilities here. One careless action at the bedside will undo hours of lecturing about the dignity of patients. Conversely, one act of kindness and consideration will make compassion a reality and an authentic experience. Student disaffection is often a masked appeal for models they can sincerely imitate.

There are some obvious critical incidents in the life of a medical student that can have a profound effect on his emotional maturation as a person.

The way the faculty handles his responses to these experiences may determine whether or not the student later approaches his own patients humanely. Some of the nodal points at which a student may need help in dealing with his own feelings are the first encounter with the cadaver or with the hopelessly ill or dying patient, the death of his "own" first patient, identifying with young patients who are seriously ill or disabled, and trying to help patients seeking assistance in the vast, impersonalized, hurried, and often physically depressing circumstances prevalent in too many large teaching hospitals.

Opportunities must be provided for students to express their feelings of conflict and anxiety with many of these potentially shattering experiences. Some personal adaptation must be effected that avoids rejection of self or profession, on the one hand, or too ready acceptance of the inevitability of an impersonal attitude, on the other. A judicious and interested faculty can encourage students to persist in gaining competence while simultaneously working to make the care of patients more humane. Even the well-intentioned student may be tempted to subvert the effort required to attain competence by self-righteous attacks on the "system" and the human failings of the clinical faculty.

Compassion and the Patient. — Humaneness and compassion in dealing with patients, the focal point of our concern, is not easily measurable. Yet, there are some rather simple behavioral criteria that can be monitored specifically as a beginning effort in any attempt to see whether at least the rudiments of humaneness and consideration are being exhibited. Clinical faculty and students might repeatedly ask themselves a series of very simple questions that arise in every patient-physician encounter.

First, do we teach students to satisfy the fundamental questions every person who is ill and anxious brings to the physician? The patient wants to know: What's wrong? How did he get that way? Is it serious? Can you cure it? What will it cost in money and loss of dignity? What are you going to do? Will it hurt? These are simple questions, but to an alarming degree, patients may see many doctors, have many tests, pay many bills, and not receive answers to these simple questions.

The issuance of a diagnosis and a standardized explanation may be convenient for the physician or all that his time will permit. Yet, this can be the first step in making the patient an object and not a person. Each patient wants answers to all these questions put into the context of his life. This is more than individual treatment, which merely means treatment as a unit. Personal treatment, instead, gets at the uniqueness of the person behind the unit. Or, as Thomas Merton said so sagely, "The person must be rescued from the individual."[5] Physicians who have neither the time nor inclination for this degree of personalization are bound by the first rule of humaneness to see that other members of the health care team are permitted to answer the personal questions that lie at the root of the patient's plea for help.

Second, can we accept the patient for what he is and not what we think he should be? The German novelist Hermann Hesse puts it well: "No man has ever been entirely and completely himself. Yet each one strives to become that — one in an awkward, the other in an intelligent way."[6] To be compassionate, we must accept each person's striving — the ignorant and the intelligent, the successes, the failures, the poor, the wise, the weak, the strong, and even the evil ones. All must receive our expression of willingness to help. This is impossible unless we continue to grow as persons ourselves. "If the doctor wants to help a human being, he must be able to accept him as he is. And he can do this in reality only when he has already seen and accepted himself as he is." We can never feel with another person when we pass superior judgment, only when we see our own frailties as well as his.

Third, do we handle our authority in a humane way that respects the life values of the patient? The health professional is always in danger of extending his authority in technical matters over the patient's system of beliefs and values. Dag Hammarskjold articulated the unique responsibility of those in authority thus: "Your position never gives you the right to command. It only imposes on you the duty of so living your life that others can receive your orders without being humiliated."[8] This is sound advice, to which we must attend whether we deal with patients, students, or our own professional colleagues. It has an important corollary: We must not "put down" the patient when he detects our uncertainties and even our errors. To be humane, we must ever be ready, as Galileo said, "to pronounce that wise, ingenious, and modest statement — 'I do not know.' "

Compassion, practiced in these terms in each individual patient transaction, is the irreducible base for mitigating the inherent dehumanizing tendencies of today's highly institutionalized and technologically oriented patterns of patient care. The student's distress with deficiencies in our present system is meaningless unless he realizes he can remedy them by humanizing his own relationships with the patients he is privileged to examine and help.

Compassion and "Humanistic" Psychology. — Recently, a variety of means derived from "humanistic" psychology have been introduced to improve the experiential-affective elements of learning. Carl Rogers has called for the use of the encounter group involving faculty and students in an attempt to forge a better unity between cognitive and affective learning. He has urged a reappraisal of all education from this point of view and has already initiated a series of encounter sessions for medical educators for this purpose.[9] Other measures, like psychodrama and psychosynthesis, are sure to be explored in an effort to remedy the defects in affective learning among medical faculty, students, and practitioners.

The success of such measures will be difficult to evaluate. For some, they will no doubt leave a lasting impression; others will reject them. For many, a transient experience of limited value will probably occur. We must avoid the conclusion that the only way to learn the affective components of humane medicine lies in any particular psychological mode. There is as much danger of psychologic overkill in medical education as there is of scientific overkill.

We cannot ignore the capacity of at least some students to become empathetic, humane, and sensitive practitioners without necessarily dissecting their emotional lives to this fine degree.

Little of a lasting nature will be achieved until the affective components in the student's learning become the conscious concern of the majority of clinical teachers. To limit this concern, and the teaching that goes with it, to those whose specialties are in psychology or the behavioral sciences is to create a pedagogic ghetto that many students and faculty will eschew.

Before they can be evaluated properly, the newer psychologic techniques must be continuing experiences for teachers and students in their own institutions. One possible achievement, as judged by my conversations with those who have attended the Rogers sessions, is a reduction in the emotional overtones that seriously impede discussions of even the cognitive elements in medical education. If encounter sessions encourage a more reasonable dialogue in the cognitive domain, they will be well worth the effort.

Affective experiences and behavioral enhancements of humane attitudes by newer psychological techniques are promising, but the affective elements in the patient-physician transaction must also be studies in an intellectually rigorous fashion. The Spanish medical philosopher Pedro Lain Entralgo has undertaken a comprehensive analysis of this subject.[10] His work is an excellent starting point for those who wish to approach the subject cognitively. Ideally, the affective training of both student and teacher should be united with the cognitive examination of the affective components in the personal relationships of patient and physician, student and teacher, and student and patient.

The Cognitive Components

The Domain of Liberal Studies. — Medical students today are, commendably, most concerned with the affective components. They exalt them, perhaps too readily, over the cognitive in their zeal to remedy some of the more obvious depersonalizing tendencies in medical education and practice. In the past, we have run the danger of suppressing the human values in medicine by an overadulation of its rational and scientific elements. We will not serve mankind any the better if we now yield to the dominance of romanticism, intuition, and introspection propounded by some under the heading of medical humanism.

As a cognitive entity, humanism has a complex history, which Kristeller and others have attempted to clarify.[11] It originated in the 19th century with Niethammer as *humanismus*, an ideal of the classical and liberal forms of education to be set against the vocational and scientific then gaining ground in education. *Humanism* itself derives from the word *umanista* used in the Italian universities of the Renaissance to designate the teachers of the humanities — those studies included in the *studia humanitatis*, the language and literature of Rome and, to a lesser extent, of Greece.

In this older sense, humanism is a literary and educational ideal, one that has lost much ground in today's universities. But almost from the outset, the term became identified with a certain set of values that set man as the central focus of concern — belief in the dignity and worth of the person, the democratic process, and human rationality. These values, as Edel has emphasized, are not a philosophical system sui generis, but rather what he terms a "philosophical strain" or "a corrective process, the guardian of a human balance against seeing man as more than a man or less than a man."[12] This "strain" is expressed in an extreme form in the religion of man proposed by Auguste Comte. More commonly, it is a bias found in many philosophical systems. Thus, we can speak of Christian, marxist, atheistic, or scientific humanisms. The humanist strain deals with values, and it is thus quite different in cognitive content from the more classical form of literary humanism.

Classical and Literary Humanism. — Let us first examine the cognitive elements in traditional or literary humanism. This ideal was best exemplified in the lives of such physician-scholars as Linacre, Caius, and their modern counterpart, Sir William Osler. Gilbert Murray said of Osler, in nominating him for the presidency of the Classical Association, that

he stands for a type of culture which the Classical Association does not wish to see die out of this world — the culture of a man who, while devoting himself to his special science, keeps nevertheless a broad basis of interest in letters of all kinds.[13]

Osler is essentially the physician as educated man, combining superb clinical talents, scientific perspective, and human concern with the capacity to excel in those skills that traditionally have been identified with a liberal education — the ability to think, write, and speak with clarity, taste, persuasiveness, and moral sensitivity. As Else has pointed out, language was the principal means through which these goals were attained.[14] These were the skills which freed man, "liberated" him, and made him human.

The cognitive skills thus subsumed in this sense of humanism were those that uniquely belong to man — the capacity to speak, write, reason, invent, create the beautiful, and judge it. Traditionally, they were taught by formal study of the disciplines of languages, literature, history, philosophy, and especially as exemplified in the writings of the Roman and Greek classics.

Education of this type is no longer a common denominator for professional people. Indeed, it is regarded by some as elitist and even antithetical to the major social responsibilities of physicians. It is, moreover, an education increasingly difficult to obtain by reason of today's crisis in the humanities. This crisis is the culmination of several factors: a decline in the teaching of the classical languages in which literary humanism is based; transformation of the humanities into technical specialties; and a decided shift in cultural ambience toward the nonliterary and more intuitive modes of communication and expression.

Genuine literary humanism has always been a rare accomplishment for physicians as for other men. Some medical educators and practitioners still persist in the hope that some formula can be found enabling us to produce physicians who are educated men in this sense, and this is essential if medicine is to be humanized. The cognitive elements of classical humanism are undeniably important for physicians as professionals; even more so if physicians are to transcend the confines of even so broad a discipline as medicine. It is as Berenson said of the Italian painters of the Renaissance, "Painting therefore offers but a partial and not always the most adequate manifestation of their personality, and we feel the artist as greater than his work, and the man as soaring above the artist."[15] The cognitive elements in literary humanism can enable the physician to "soar above" his profession.

Not many students today perceive the value of a rigorous education in the cognitive elements of traditional humanism. Some will perceive them later in life, when medicine itself becomes so routinized as to verge on boredom.

Others, perhaps the majority, will never perceive the life-enhancing qualities of traditional humanistic study. What, then, is a realistic future for the cognitive skills and knowledge supposedly imparted by liberal studies in the education of physicians?

Humanities in Medicine: Approach for Today. — We cannot permit the possibility of contact with traditional humanism to decay completely. Too much of man's capacity for a life of satisfaction is contained within it. We owe every student at least the opportunity for contact with liberal studies at some point in his education. But today we are required to offer this opportunity in a variety of ways not limited to the premedical years.

Some students will continue to follow the pattern of a professional education built on a prior base in the liberal arts. For the majority, the most effective teaching of humanistic studies will occur within the context of medical education itself. Here, the student's motivation and goal directedness will help to focus the cognitive features of the humanities. The medical context is rich in possibilities for explicating the essential cognitive skills unique to humane and liberal studies. The pedagogic aim in the predegree years is to uncover the student's interest in these skills and, in the years of continuing education, to reinforce them in his own experiences as a person dealing with other persons in the medical transaction.

This mode of teaching the cognitive components of humanism will require special adaptations of *what* is to be taught, *how* it is taught, and *who* teaches it. At this time, a variety of approaches is being tried in a dozen or so medical institutions attempting to infuse humanistic elements into the corpus of medical education. Two recent institutes on this subject, under the auspices of the Society for Health and Human Values, summarize these current experiments.[16] While these reports indicate a wide range of approaches, some conclusions seem quite clear.

First, what is to be learned? There is no one discipline or combination of disciplines that will assure acquisition of the requisite intellectual skills. Instead, what we must seek is to inculcate that knowledge an educated man must have to distinguish him from his colleagues who are merely competent. Professor Wayne Booth succinctly summarizes these skills as learning how to think critically for ourselves, how to experience beauty for ourselves, and to make our own choices among possible actions.[17] These are the skills that make a man free — the "liberal arts." If he possesses them, he is no longer subservient to the thoughts, actions, or esthetics of those who can examine these matters critically. Neither the sciences nor the humanities can encompass these skills entirely. Each can contribute to their development. The traditional emphasis on the literary content of the humanities must be expanded to include some of what the scientist now contributes to our cultural milieu.

Second, how shall these skills be taught? To be most effective with the goal-oriented medical student, the cognitive skills should be taught within the framework of a medical education — indeed, as an integral part of that education. Medicine is admirably suited to this purpose. It abounds in experiential data about the human condition and illustrates easily the concrete importance of the cognitive skills of humanism in clinical decision-making, the lack of which, in my opinion, is one of the major defects of clinical medicine today. Medicine is also the focal point for much of our most recent and important knowledge of man and his behavior.

Teaching in such a context necessarily proceeds from the concrete, personal, and immediate to the abstract, general, and more ultimate concerns of mankind. It demands use of the case method and seminar rather than the lecture and reading assignment. It centers on personal involvement by the student with the specific concerns of his patient and thus gains a relevance scarcely equalled in other types of teaching.

These teaching modes are quite unfamiliar to the usual teacher of the humanities, and this brings us to our last question: Who shall teach? Certain special characteristics are demanded of the teacher who essays to teach the cognitive skills of humanism in the medical setting. He must be an able and secure scholar in his own discipline; he must be committed to communicating that discipline to medical students and physicians; and he must be willing to enter serious and continuing dialogue with the medical culture, while bringing his special viewpoint to bear on the phenomena of the medical experience.

Not many bona fide humanists are prepared for this sort of teaching. Hopefully, more of them will see challenges and benefits for their own studies in an intimate exchange with medicine. If current interest among medical educators grows, we will need to educate some humanists specifically for the engagement with medicine. There is some danger at present, as with any new field as yet unproven intellectually, that the field may fall to the willing and eager rather than to the most competent teachers.

Clearly, the cognitive components of traditional humanism embracing its literary elements and its intellectual attitudes are important in the education of the physician-humanist. To be effective and useful in today's university and with today's student requires a mode of teaching and a faculty with characteristics different from those that prevail in the universities' departments of humanities at present.[18] [19]

The Domain of Values. — There is another domain of cognitive knowledge that is contained in the concept of the humanist-physician, and that is the domain of values as objects of serious study in medical education. We cannot provide medical care within a humanist frame without a knowledge of the intersections in values that occur at every stage of the medical transaction. The meanings of these intersections for the patient, the physician, and society bear directly on the outcome of medical management. Medical teaching now requires the infusion of a perception of the value questions as a correlative device, much in the spirit of the humanistic strain alluded to by Edel.[12]

At every step in the medical encounter, human values are set against each other: those of the patient with those of the physician, those of society with those of the individual, and those of the physician as scientist and teacher with those of the physician as healer. Each person and each community is identified by commitment to a certain configuration of beliefs, choices, and priorities about the things believed to be important. These values have meanings quite specific for each person and each community, and these meanings must be understood by anyone who presumes to treat either the person or the community.

We now live in an era in which the ancient and long-standing image of the physician as a benign authoritarian is intolerable to most educated people. Patients have the right to make choices among alternative modes of management in keeping with the values they conceive to be most important to them. The physician must understand the basis of the patient's value choices, respect them, and work within their confines much more sensitively than ever before. In a matter so personal as health, the imposition of one person's values over another's — even of the physician's over the patient's — is a moral injustice.

Practitioners, students, and faculty members, therefore, need a formal knowledge of the meaning of values and the varieties of systems within which values are expressed. They need especially to understand the genesis of their own value systems and to recognize the gap that inevitably develops between the values of the professional and those of the society within which a profession may function.

Physicians do not reflect very often on the values peculiar to the process of professionalization through which they pass. Nor are they and their teachers sufficiently conscious of the imprint made by the prevailing mode of medical education and its traditional orientation on their own value systems. These values very soon become the prelogical foundations for the physician's behavior, for his normative ethics, and for his apodictic statements on what is good for the patient and society.

The significance of an orientation to values as objects of more serious study and experience in medical education is very much heightened by the new problems of individual and social ethics which derive from the enhanced capabilities of modern biomedical science.[20] The physician's stance with reference to abortion, euthanasia, human experimentation, genetic manipulation, behavioral control, and a variety of other urgent and dramatic new issues in medical practice is based in a set of values the foundations of which he rarely examines critically.

It is impossible to confront these and other new questions in the ethics of health care without a reconceptualization of the foundations of medical ethics. Such a restructuring of traditional normative and deontological ethics is dependent on a reconceptualization of the values on which traditional and contemporary ethics systems are based. Value questions underlie the legal, political, and social mechanisms for decision-making in the public as well as the most private matters of medical and health care.

Medical axiology is an underdeveloped — indeed, almost nonexistent — discipline at this time. It can be taught at several levels — at the fundamental level of value theory, then at the applied level of clinical decision-making, and finally at the community level of public policy-making. Integration of knowledge from a variety of disciplines is requisite if a true medical axiology is to emerge. Law, ethics, political science, philosophy, and social and cultural anthropology are intermingled in any critical inquiry into the value questions in health care.

"Medical" axiology, like "medical" philosophy, "medical" history, or "medical" sociology, demands an interdigitation of principles from the humanities and the social sciences with the concrete experiential data derived from specific clinical situations in which value questions influence the outcome for human beings seeking help. A whole new set of questions of very great human concern is emanating from the emerging dialogue between medicine and biology, on the one hand, and various of the humanities and social sciences, on the other.

These questions at the interzone between medicine and the other university disciplines have not been explored in depth. Yet, even at this early stage, they must be taught and exemplified in medical education. The content and the methods requisite to teaching at the junctions of medicine, the humanities, and the social sciences are just beginning to receive explicit attention.[16] No success-assured formula is available for wide application. The impatient student who hopes to humanize medicine overnight through some curricular thaumaturgy is sure to be disappointed.

In the immediate future, we face a tense period in our attempts to develop a more humanistic frame for medical education. On the one hand, our knowledge of human values is rudimentary and needs deepening. On the other, we face the urgency and the high expectations of all who hope for elimination of the deficiencies in our present modes of learning. Faculties in medicine and in the traditional disciplines must undergo significant attitudinal adjustments before these nascent studies can flourish. Concomitantly, they must also develop the intellectual rigor without which they cannot survive in the medical curriculum.

Nevertheless, the formal teaching of human values, at all levels of medical education, offers a sound mechanism for liberalizing and humanizing the student's technical and professional learning. The study of values may well provide a more realistic and a more widely applicable avenue for liberal education for today's medical students than the cognitive elements of traditional or literary humanism. Without deprecating the latter, it seems more likely that the study of human values will open a more attractive road toward attainment of those attitudes of mind formerly associated with the best in traditional humanistic studies.

It goes without saying that learning the cognitive domain of human values will be totally ineffectual if it is not accompanied by affective learning and by explicit example in the behavior of the faculty, especially its clinical members. In the realm of values, the humanistic strain is attainable only where the patient is in fact treated with full dignity as a man, enabled to participate democratically in decisions that affect his being, and approached with tolerance for his fallibility and that of his physician.

The Ideal Resynthesized

For the purposes of clarification of the goals of his education, we have intentionally disassembled the ideal of the humanist-physician. This disassembly enables us to understand the full spectrum of meanings within the ideal and to denote educational goals specifically designed to explicate each of the integral components of humanism. By so doing, we can avoid diffusing our educational goals over a vague territory more emotionally than rationally defined. More important, our dissection may perhaps permit a resynthesis of the ideal in terms more consistent with the motivations of today's students and the contemporary responsibilities of the profession.

The ideal humanist-physician would fuse all elements — the affective and the cognitive domains we have described — the whole built on a base of technical competence. Professional education, then, has as its goal the making of a competent clinical craftsman; affective learning has the goal of making a humane and compassionate practitioner; and the cognitive elements of humanism, modified in the two ways I have suggested, should make for an educated practitioner. These three levels in the life of the physician should interpenetrate and reinforce each other. Very few persons will ever experience excellence in all dimensions, but recognition of the full expression of the ideal establishes a bench mark against which the degree of an individual's humanistic education can be assessed.

Medicine enjoys a special position among the disciplines. It centers on man in all his dimensions and shares some part of his reality with the humanities, the social sciences, and the experimental sciences. Pursued to its fullest expression, medicine can be truly humanizing, for its object of study and concern is man.

John Ciardi's recent exposition of the concept of esthetic wisdom is apposite: "the sum total of all the great artist becomes in his life's exposure to his medium. The artist's environment," he adds, "is not the world but the world as his medium reveals it."[21]

I submit that medicine, like the arts, also provides a kind of human experience that makes it a special medium for revealing the world. It, too, can yield an esthetic wisdom of its own special object, man. Medicine taught in a humanistic frame prepares the student for its humane practice. Practice in a humanistic frame reveals even more about the microcosm, as Caraka perceived in the quotation that opened this essay.

FOOTNOTES

1. *The Caraka Samhita*. S. Gulabkunverba (trans), Jamnagar, India, Ayurvedic Society, 1949, vol 1, p 469.
2. Aulus Gellius, cited by Crane RS: *The Idea of the Humanities and Other Essays Critical and Historical*. Chicago, University of Chicago Press, 1968, p 23.
3. Pellegrino ED: The non-Renaissance man. *Pharos of Alpha Omega Alpha* 32 (No. 1): 16-17, 1969.
4. Jung C: *Psychological Reflections*. J. Jacobi (ed), Princeton, NJ, Bollingen Series XXI, 1970, p 84.
5. Merton T: *New Seeds of Contemplation*. New York, New Directions, 1961, p 38.
6. Hesse H: *Demian*. New York, Bantam Books Inc, 1970, prologue.
7. Jung C: *Psychological Reflections*. J. Jacobi (ed), Princeton, NJ, Bollington Series XXI, 1970, p 90.
8. Hammarskjold D: *Markings*. New York, Alfred A. Knopf Inc, 1965, p 105.
9. Rogers C: Bringing together ideas and feeling in learning. *Learning Today* 5 (No. 2): 32-43, 1972.
10. Entralgo PL: *La Relacion Medico-Enfermo Historia y Teoria*. Madrid, Revista de Occidente, 1964.
11. Kristeller PO: *Renaissance Thought: The Classic and Scholastic and Humanist Strains*. New York, Harper Torchbooks 1961, pp 8-23.
12. Edel A: Where is the crisis in humanism? *Rev Int Philosophie*, fasc 3-4, 1968, pp 284-295.
13. Murray G, quoted by Cushing H: *Introduction to Sir William Osler: The Old Humanities and the New Science*. Boston, Houghton Mifflin Co, 1920, p x.
14. Else G: The old and the new humanities. *Daedalus* 98:803-804, 1969.
15. Berenson B: *Italian Painters of the Renaissance: Florentine and Central Italian Schools*. New York, Phaidon, 1968, vol 2, p 1.
16. *Proceedings of the Institute on Human Values in Medicine*. Philadelphia, Society for Health and Human Values, 1972, vol 2, pp BP 1-BP 83.
17. Booth W: Is there any knowledge that a man must have? in WC Booth (ed): *The Knowledge Most Worth Having*. Chicago, University of Chicago Press, 1967, pp i-28.
18. Pellegrino ED: The most humane science: Some notes on liberal education in medicine and the university, the sixth Sanger lecture. *Bull Med Col Va* 2:11-39, 1970.
19. Pellegrino ED: Reflections, refractions, and prospectives, in *Proceedings of the Institute on Human Values in Medicine*. Philadelphia, Society for Health and Human Values, 1972, vol 1, pp 99-115.

SECTION 5

Seeds of Contemplation

Introduction

An examination of the contemporary issues and trends which are of pervasive importance in the health field are presented in this section. The new directions and major thrusts which are examined in our three selections reflect the dynamic environment in which the health system operates. A careful deliberation of these trends will sharpen the meaning of our humanistic perceptions and guide the patterns of action that we choose to achieve our humanistic objective. To meet and maintain this objective, we must attempt to develop a consistent orientation to the changing environment of the future. If we identify, and forecast, the social, political, and economic health trends, we will be in a better position to deal with and influence the inherent challenges, opportunities, and obstacles which these trends create.

Our concluding section begins with a selection by David Hayes-Bautista and Dominic S. Harveston, "Holistic Health Care." Holistic Health is a term being used currently to describe concepts and practices in health care that transcend or radically alter current health care practices. The content and linkage of these concepts and practices have profound implications for the health system.

A unique and significant analysis of quality of care evaluation is presented in our second selection, "Measuring and Evaluating Hospital and Medical Care" by Avedis Donobedian. Increasing attention is being paid to the problems of defining, improving and appraising quality of care. It is difficult to define; it is complex and elusive to measure. Quality, though elusive, is not an abstraction. In the first part of his essay, Donobedian observes that "we, who are unable to decide how best to assess the quality of the technical management of physical-physiological illness, shall be required, first, to determine criteria and standards for social and psychological management and, second, to resolve the ethical dilemmas of reconciling the interests of the individual patient with those of the collectivity — the heart of resource allocation. But we have no choice. We must venture forth."

A critical and agonizing indictment of our current health care system is presented in our concluding and provocative selection, "Medical Nemesis" by Ivan Illich. Illich is greatly concerned about the need to change our consciousness of and our ways of thinking about health and health care. Illich's polemic essay is a substantial contribution to the ongoing dialogue that is essential to progress in the health care system.

Holistic Health Care

David Hayes-Bautista and Dominic S. Harveston

In the past decade a great number of alternative health-care delivery centers have opened without the blessings of organized medicine. The exact number of these centers is not known, and given the rather short lives of many such centers, their number will probably remain unknown. They do, however, represent an interesting and important phenomenon which deserves to be studied.

A most useful way of approaching the study of this rather amorphous grouping of alternative health-care delivery systems is to conceptualize them as a social movement (Hayes-Bautista, 1976). As noted by Haberle (1951), one of the first steps to be taken in understanding a social movement is an exposition of the content of the ideology upon which it is based. Community clinics have an ideology which does make them a legitimate object of study as a social movement. Like most social movements, however, this ideology is not well formalized. The purpose of this paper is to begin to formalize community clinic ideology, to locate it historically within the context of other health-based social movements (Hayes-Bautista, 1976), and then to examine the policy implications of the new definitions of health, illness, and society that have emerged with it.

Pathogenic Location

We will use the concept of *pathogenic location* to describe different institutional approaches to health and illness behavior. By determining an institution's view of the pathogenic location, we may gain a rapid summary of that organization's notion of what constitutes medical reality.

Briefly defined, the pathogenic location refers to where one places the ultimate origin of health and illness between two end points of a continuum: the location inside the individual at a microbiological level, and the location outside the individual in the ecosphere. We shall look at the end points of this continuum, the basic underlying concepts and history of each, review how these conceptual underpinnings influence the behavior and organization of a community clinic, and then discuss policy problems.

The Medical Model

The medical model forms the conceptual basis for most current efforts in medical care in this country. This rather recent view of illness causation (only a century old) has had tremendous impact on health policy in this country. As many community clinics are opposed to a strict application of

From *Journal of Social Policy*, Vol. 7, No. 5, March/April 1977. By permission of the authors and publisher, Social Policy Corporation, New York, New York 10036.
Copyright © 1977 by Social Policy Corporation.

the medical model and attendant policies, it will be useful to see what this conceptual basis refers to.

In terms of the pathogenic location, the medical model places the ultimate origin of illness inside the individual, at a microbiological level. Efforts may then be concentrated at that level, and such efforts are based on the following assumptions:

1. An illness has an organic base (Veatch, 1973).
2. The organic base is the result of discrete causal elements (Dubos, 1959).
3. The illness is the involuntary result of an invasion of the host by an overwhelming quantity of the causal element (Veatch, 1973).
4. The appropriate treatment for an illness is an agent which will directly counterattack the causal element and neutralize it (Dubos, 1959).
5. Such an agent can be prescribed and administered only by a technically competent specialist (Parsons, 1951; Veatch, 1973).
6. The knowlege held by the specialist is inaccessible to the layperson, hence the patient must submit to the ministrations of the specialist without interference (Parsons, 1951; R. Blum, 1960).

When this set of assumptions becomes the lens through which the world is viewed, certain types of actions are suggested and reinforced, while others are rejected or ignored. These assumptions have formed a formal, explicit ideology and have given rise to behaviors which have become institutionalized. The weight and inertia of these institutions tend to entrench this ideology, and have forced others out of the marketplace of ideas.

One of the first results of this ideology was the focusing of attention at the microbiological level, whereas at other times it has been placed at an extraindividual level. In order to better handle and control events, the individual has been divided into turfs, each the province of a set of specialists who feature increasing knowledge about a single organ, single tissue, single cell, and single procedure (H. Blum, 1975). This ideology serves as the underpinning and impetus for the development of actions which form the functional basis of a kind of medical care which deals on a fragmented basis with fragments of an individual (Simon, 1961). The whole individual and the society in which he/she operates are lost in a welter of organs, tissues, cells, bacteria, and procedures.

A second result of this approach to the world is that if a state of being does not fit or cannot be fitted into the above set of assumptions of the medical model, it is declared to be something other than a medical problem (H. Blum, 1975; Dubos, 1959).

A third result of this ideology is a tendency to redefine social problems (such as alcoholism, drug use, juvenile delinquency) as medical problems. This translates symptoms into clinical concepts which physicians can manage. Once so defined, effort may be expended for the discovery of the appropriate neutralizing agent (in the problems above, Antabuse, Methadone and Ritalin, respectively, are used). By so "medicalizing" social problems, they can become the province of medical care (Bernstein & Lennard, 1973; Freidson, 1970; Ehrenreich & Ehrenreich, 1974).

The Holistic Health Model

While the medical model has been fairly well developed formally, the ideologies of the new community clinics have not been given as much attention. By use of the pathogenic location conceptualization, we shall now see what some of these ideologies are and attempt to give form to some of the underlying notions of what constitutes appropriate health-care activities.

In contrast to the medical model, in the holistic model the pathogenic location is placed outside the individual. This placement implies that attention and activity must be concentrated on units larger than the individual. While not rejecting the notion that there are microbiological elements involved in illness, the holistic model also includes and places attention upon causal elements which are often political, economic, social, and psychological as well. All of these elements must be addressed, and no illness is "cured" until the root cause elements have been successfully dealt with. With this idea comes the notion that if attention is focused only upon the somatic level, health will never be achieved, although illness might be occasionally and temporarily controlled. Placing the pathogenic location outside the individual appears to lead to the following assumptions about health-care activities:

Individual illness is a reflection of societal illness. It is assumed in this model that the conditions external to an individual are (or can be) under societal control. In this fashion, then, an ill society will yield naught but ill individuals. Economic woes, cultural dislocations, racial strife, and inadequate housing are examples of nonmicrobiological elements which would have to be addressed in a holistic treatment before any related illness in an individual could be said to be cured.

Multiple causation. By expanding the scope to include conditions external to an individual, the holistic model brings in many nonmicrobiological facets of an illness. Among some of those of current interest to community clinics are: unemployment, racism, malnutrition, education, housing, urban congestion, pollution, and overly stressful living patterns and working conditions. Any or all of these facets may be as important as the organic ones.

Multiple interventions. Given the notion of multiple causation, a community clinic must then embark upon a set of multiple, simultaneous measures in order to achieve health for a population. There are two levels of multiple interventions such clinics must keep in mind: the individual and the institutional. First, regarding the individual level, many clinics operate on the notion that multiple causation is not confined to the world outside an individual, but may very well be operating within an individual. Thus, many clinics offer multiple treatment options. Some of these are fairly standard, such as the offering of psychological services along with medical ones. Often, however, clinics will attempt to gather radically different healing options which are not usually sanctioned by medicine, such as chiropractors, acupuncturists, folk healers, spiritual healers, meditation therapies, natural foods, postural integration, and others which are currently in vogue.

On the other hand, when the pathogenic location view demonstrates that some of the main causal elements of an illness are outside an individual, a community clinic may desire to take action at an institutional level. Quite often this means that the community clinic will have to act on behalf of a patient or a number of patients as a patient advocate or health ombudsperson to the established health institutions of a community. This also extends beyond the health institutions to agencies, establishments, or organizations which create unhealthy situations and cause illness. In these cases the community clinic may find itself involved in political action.

Curative care is ultimately insufficient. If the pathogenic location is more often outside the individual than within, it makes little sense to "cure" the individual only to send her/him back into the same society and environment which caused the condition in the first place. The patient will simply return at a later date for more individual "cure". In this respect, much current medical care effort in this country is seen as band-aid attempts, effecting only superficial cure and not dealing with the deep-rooted causal agents.

Once a state of health is achieved, it requires active effort to be maintained. The job of health-care institutions should then be twofold: to raise the level of health by active intervention and environmental and institutional manipulation, and then, by active effort, to maintain that level of health in its service population.

Social restructuring is necessary to effectively achieve and maintain an acceptable level of health. The amount of restructuring needed will vary from asking for minor changes in existing institutions and relationships to demanding a complete rebuilding of society as it is currently known.

A Classification Scheme

We can now examine an institution's adherence to the notion of holistic health by classifying according to where the locus of the cause and cure of illness is to be found. In the medical model the locus is in the microbiological area: in essence, everyone is assumed to be well, and deviance is introduced by a massive invasion of an organism by foreign agents that is beyond the individual's capacity to resist. The responsibility of medical care, then, is to heal individuals so that they can return to their normal places in society and fulfill their functions until another bout of illness makes such operation nonfunctional once again. The sick role (Parsons, 1951; Gordon, 1966) has often been used to epitomize this process: a sick person is separated from society, made well, then placed back into society as a functioning unit.

In the holistic health model, the locus of causation and cure is enlarged to include the society at large. In a holistic sense, making an individual well is ultimately self-defeating if that individual is placed back into the same type of situation that caused the illness initially. It is the responsibility of an institution to heal not only the individual, but also the society which creates

FIGURE 1

MEDICAL MODEL

Look for illness and health at micro-biological level. Heal individual to return to normal functions in society.

HOLISTIC HEALTH MODEL

Look for illness and health at the societal level. Question if society is structured to provide a healthful living environment. An ill society will produce ill members.

FIGURE 2

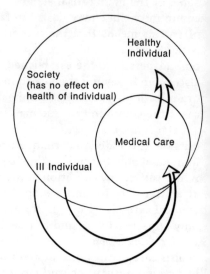

FIGURE 3

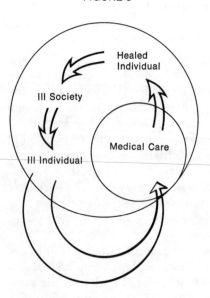

FIGURE 4

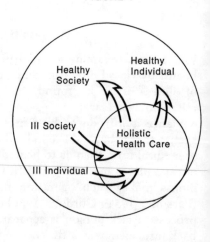

the sick individual. Many clinics further take the position that society must be healed before an individual can begin to think about health.

Thus we have our first paradigm, which can be visualized as a continuum with the medical model and the holistic health model as the two end points. As in most paradigms, few institutions would achieve the end points; most would be clustered at different locations along this continuum.

An alternative way of looking at this paradigm is seen in Figures 2, 3, and 4. Figure 2 is a representation of the process of medical care as envisioned by the medical model. The first important assumption is the pathogenic location. Illness is located within an individual, and the surrounding society has very little, if anything, to do with the occurrence of illness. If society does appear to have an effect, dealing with it is not within the purview of medical care. An individual becomes ill due to some individual failing, is removed from society by the medical care process, healed, then placed back in society. It is assumed that an individual will remain healthy until there is a recurrence of some sort of individual failure.

Figure 3 represents a community clinic's view of the actual effects of standard medical model treatment. Here, the pathogenic location is placed outside the organism. Thus, a society creates illness in its individuals. If they are removed, healed, and placed back in society, the individual will become ill once again. In one sense, such a view contends that society itself is suffering from illnesses of various sorts, which are manifested in individual members' illnesses.

Figure 4 shows an ideal model of holistic health action. Both the individual and the society are fit patients for the ministrations of holistic health care. Together, ill individual and society are made healthy, and positive actions are taken later to maintain that health level. In this view the need for curative medical care is reduced due to lessened demand.

A History of Conflicting Policies

By using the ideal types which are the end points of the pathogenic location continuum, we notice that there are two basic ideologies which can direct and control health-care activities. While there is no logical reason for these to be mutually exclusive, in the past and in the present this has often been the case with respect to health policies. In ancient Greece, Panacea was the healing goddess (with whom the medical model can be in part identified) while Hygea was the goddess of health achieved through appropriate living (with whom the holistic health model can be identified) (Dubos, 1959). Translated into policy, ancient Greece was the scene of conflict between physicians who were curatively oriented in their approach to health and philosophers who felt that much of the physician's mystical knowledge kept people, particularly the poor who could not pay for physicians' services, from achieving good health (Edelstein, 1967).

More recently, the precursors of the public health movements in Europe and the United States have had to deal with the dichotomy between the medical and holistic models of health-care actions. Chadwick, writing of the mortality rates among the urban poor of England in 1842, did not have the germ theory in hand to explain why poorer people were dying at an earlier age than rural landed gentry (average age at death for laborers in Manchester was 17, while for gentry in Rutlandshire it was 51). Because he could not focus on a single causal agent, he was forced to develop a holistic approach in which he identified the social milieu in general as the causal condition. For example, Chadwick (1842) noticed that the incidence of tuberculosis increased with certain social conditions: overcrowding, poverty, high birthrates, alcoholism, and malnutrition. The "cure" he proposed for tuberculosis was not a chemoprophylaxis to arrest development of the tubercle bacillus (which would be based on the medical model), but rather a provision for social reform: construction of adequate housing with proper ventilation, provision of jobs, education, sanitation, etc. (Chadwick, 1887). Shattuck, writing later in Boston and heavily influenced by Chadwick, arrived at similar conclusions for similar reasons: unable to point to a single causal agent, he described a multiplicity of them, most of which had their roots in the social and environmental order of an area (Shattuck, 1948).

One of the most striking proponents of the holistic approach to medical care in the pre-germ theory phase was Virchow, who in 1848 considered physicians to be the natural attorneys of the poor (Kroeger, 1937) and went so far as to state that "medicine is a social science and politics nothing but medicine on a grand scale" (Rosen, 1974; p. 62). Believing that medicine should intervene in political and social life in order to accomplish its purpose, Virchow developed the theory that social and cultural maladjustments occasioned by the massive shifts of labor forces from rural to urban areas were manifested in epidemic diseases (Rosen, 1974). A contemporary of Virchow, Neumann, singled out not physical conditions of an individual, but social conditions as the primary cause of premature death (Kroeger, 1937).

Thus, the initial thrust of the public health movement was toward a holistic notion of the pathogenic location, placing the cause outside the individual and recognizing that there were often multiple causes.

Unwittingly, Pasteur created the shift from the holistic approach to health to the medical model. Thanks to his ceaseless curiosity, and against the opinion of many of the foremost medical experts of the day, Pasteur was able to demonstrate the existence of germs and correlate their presence with disease. After a period of resistance in the late 1860s, the great explanatory power of the medical model caught the medical world by storm, and shortly the holistic model was ridiculed as a passé, romantic, naive notion of disease causation. Yet, Pasteur, almost alone among bacteriologists who made great discoveries in the microbiological realm, still emphasized the need to not limit one's view to the strict medical model, but to consider a person in relation to his or her environment.

While Virchow was waging a losing battle against the adoption of the germ theory as the *only* cause of illness, a number of other events occurred which reinforced one another and eventually led to adoption of the germ theory throughout the American medical care world. Medical schools were being reformed along the lines of the German models which were based largely upon a mastery of the new germ theory. As a result of the Flexner report in 1910, medical schools in the United States either adopted the germ theory and related biological sciences as a basic paradigm or lost their accreditation. The growing tide of professionalism, begun with establishment of the American Medical Association, was abetted by the adoption of the germ theory, which provided a rational and tangible basis for explanation of the profession's responsibilities. As the twentieth century wore on, various governmental and private programs were developed which made use of the tremendous advances made possible by the research in the microbiological areas. Medicine came to be the province of a small group of specialists whose attention was focused upon subhuman elements.

The result has been an interlocking of interests which ties together governmental programs, medical education, research, and industry (Ehrenreich & Ehrenreich, 1970). These linkages provide a tremendous momentum in favor of the germ theory approach to medicine. Currently, most medical care policy on federal, state and local levels is tied to the medical model paradigm: accreditations, licenses, insurance, payment schedules, and organization plans are largely based upon the search for health at a microorganismic level.

Public health activities have also largely concentrated on, and been rationalized by, the search for microbiological causation, effectively placing the pathogenic location in the medical model. The emphasis has also often been upon the discovery of the appropriate "cure" which may be administered to an individual via a shot, drug, or a pill (Bernstein & Lennard, 1973).

The Academic Approach

During the eras of great microbiological discoveries and inventions of wonder drugs, it may have appeared that health could be achieved through continuous application of the medical model. Recently there has been serious concern on two levels about the limitations of that model. As we have seen, community clinics stress that health-care activities must include serious dosages of economic, social, and political action as well as strictly medical curative action. This particular wave of support for a holistic approach to health might be considered a lay movement, given that most community clinics are, or feel that they should be, under control of community members rather than health professionals.

The second locus of concern is the academic community. While Dubos was among the first to stimulate the upsurge of interest in holistic health which has been taking place on general campuses and in medical schools for the past two decades, his basic concerns have been amplified by epidemiologists who have discovered that the major killers in modern

American society are not amenable to control by simplistic application of the medical model. Indeed, these new epidemics require a more sophisticated, complex, multifaceted, and multidisciplinary approach (Winkelstein, 1972; Fuchs, 1966). The basic academic paradigm for developing a holistic approach to health has evolved out of the systems approach (Churchman, 1968). Brody (1973) has done seminal work in developing a systems view of health which holds that a person has to be viewed as the concatenation of a number of different levels of systems ranging from subatomic particles to the biosphere. A disturbance at any one level may be manifested in another level; yet the "real" cure will not be accomplished at the manifest level but rather at the level which originally contained the disturbance. Thus, if lead poisoning becomes manifest at the organic level, organ level intervention will not cure it. The level of causation is the social, political, and economic plane, and cures must be effected there. The systems paradigm has served as an intellectual underpinning for much current thought about holistic health (H. Blum, 1974; Duhl, 1975; Lynn, 1969).

Problems in Practicing Holistic Health Care

With the energies of community clinics invested more in the practice of health care than in theorizing about it, and clinic service providers and academicians doing research in the area often at a considerable remove from each other, certain problems have arisen in applying the holistic model. Below we discuss some of the major obstacles encountered by clinics.

Definition of a "holistic health problem." While it is nearly axiomatic that a problem must be fairly well defined before any sort of answer can be attempted, community clinics often find themselves in the bind of attempting to find a solution to a problem which has not yet been well thought out. Just what exactly are the holistic limits of any given health problem? While both Virchow and Neumann repeatedly stated that medicine was a social science, they both knew that much investigative work had to be done in order to understand what was meant by that. Thus, while they could observe that social and economic conditions had an effect on health and disease, the relations had to be further investigated in a scientific fashion. Only then could remedies be developed on a sound basis. Today, the notion of holistic health is not clearly understood, with the result that a clinic often has only a vague notion of what it should be addressing itself to. With holistic health problems so ill-defined, some clinics may tend to follow medical model practice simply because it does offer some definitions and the promise of conclusive action.

Lack of appropriate treatment actions. Given the diffuse nature of attempting to define health problems holistically, community clinics are often equally lacking in procedural knowledge about how to remedy that problem.

If a person comes into a community clinic with an infection, there is a set of definitions and treatment procedures to handle it on a medical model basis. Yet, how should that same problem be handled holistically? There is nothing comparable to the Physicians' Desk Reference to follow for procedure.

Personnel. Given the problems of defining and addressing a problem, next comes the question of who is to do this. Currently medical personnel are not trained to analyze a problem holistically, so that their input, while necessary, is not sufficient. Often a clinic will have to utilize a combination of physicians, nurses, attorneys, psychologists, and administrators to develop an appropriate intervention at the appropriate level. And because the practitioners of these different skills have rarely been educated to work together on a complex health problem, much time is lost in trying to figure out exactly what they should do. For example, if an area is plagued with high unemployment, some of the operational questions are: Should this be defined as a health problem? Who should reasonably be expected to handle this: the clinic, a state employment agency, a school district, a union, groupings of employers? If the clinic is to tackle the problem itself, who within it has the time and expertise to do something? Or, if the clinic is to manipulate another institution so that it, rather than the clinic, will address the health problem, who should do the manipulating, and how is that to be accomplished? Should the clinic concentrate its efforts on an individual case-by-case basis with one individual linked to one job, or should it ignore the immediate needs of individuals to work on long-term activity which will benefit more individuals at a later date? The concept of a health advocate has been mentioned as some Jack or Jill-of-all-trades who will be able to function at an individual and institutional level, who will possess medical, legal, political, and social skills, but we have yet to develop a program to train such a person.

There appear to be at least two major types of reasons for a professional's choice of work in a community clinic: ideological and political reasons, which lead to a professional consciously attempting to transcend the medical model paradigm, and personal and ethnic identity reasons in which one chooses to work with a particular group without always realizing that to do so will require new frames of reference. Once in a community clinic, health professionals are faced with opposite forces, some of which push them towards the practice of holistic health while others simultaneously pull them away from it. The forces toward the practice have largely to do with the governance: most community clinics have as one of their tenets the deprofessionalization and demystification of medical care and health care.

Thus, policy decisions may be affected by nonprofessional staff and, in many cases, by a lay governing board. With this expanded input many concerns, such as employment, education, and housing, are raised and at times made a part of a clinic's activities as well as the more purely clinical concerns. However, the forces which pull a professional away from such practice arise due to the limited amount of time, energy, and resources available to meet health care problems of great magnitude. Because medical care is needed often immediately and urgently, and because other action is often slow to have effect, many professionals find themselves practicing standard medical care in spite of their wishes and those of other policy makers in the institution.

Financing. When a community clinic decides to devote a substantial portion of its time to the delivery of holistic health, this often means the clinic must engage in activities which are not recognized by financial policy makers. Reimbursements for medical care via intermediaries (Medicaid, Medicare, private insurance) are often based upon the medical model, with the result that activities which do not fall within that model are not reimbursed. Medicaid, for example, will not reimburse a community clinic for its efforts to persuade a county board of supervisors to rezone an area so that an industry may be either attracted or repelled (depending upon that industry's relation to the health of an area). Most community clinics are in financial straits given that as a matter of course they prefer not to charge patients or to charge token amounts. Thus patient fees cannot finance the clinic's activities and other sources of revenue will not do so.

Limited resources. An additional impediment to a clinic's ability to take holistic action is limited resources. As must be apparent by now, a holistic approach is more easily preached than practiced. Because of difficulty in defining a problem, developing a set of procedures, allocating personnel, and financing the action, the holistic aspects of treatment are often given secondary importance by necessity rather than design. A holistic approach demands great amounts of time and energy, yet is not reimbursable by most current policies. It is not unusual for a community clinic to find after a period of time that its words and actions are at odds. Although desiring to deliver holistic health care, it winds up being able to deliver only medical care, with the added dimension that it is certain that those current activities are bound to be counterproductive in the long run. The decision to deliver medical care while promising health care is not made by a community clinic alone. Often patients will demand medical care, unwilling to wait for the long-term, not quite tangible benefits of holistic health action. A mother who brings an infant in pain to a community clinic wants that pain halted, not some future promise of a lawsuit designed to avoid recurrences of that pain.

For all the reasons given above, many community clinics find that they must devote substantial portions of their time to delivering medical care rather than holistic health care. Yet they are not to be blamed for failing to attain their stated goals. The fact that they recognize that they are practicing band-aid medicine places them on the path to holistic medicine. However, it is important to keep in mind that these clinics will most likely not be successful without changes in the education of health professionals and in the financing of care. Until then, holistic health actions will always be an afterthought made possible by some person's spare time, energy, and money.

BIBLIOGRAPHY

Bernstein, Arnold and Lennard, Henry L.
1973 "The American Way of Drugging: Drugs, Doctors and Junkies," *Transaction/Society* 10:14-25.

Blum, Henrik
1974   *Planning for Health.* New York: Human Sciences Press.
1975   "Factors in the Health Care Delivery System Inhibiting Utilization and What Can Be Done about Them." Berkeley: University of California, mimeo.

Blum, Richard.
1960   *The Managment of the Doctor Patient Relationship.* New York: McGraw-Hill.

Brody, Howard.
1973   "The System's View of Man: Implications for Science, Medicine and Ethics," *Perspectives in Biology and Medicine* (Autumn): 71-92.

Chadwick, Sir Edwin.
1842   *Poor Law Commissioners on an Inquiry into the Sanitary Condition of the Labouring Population of Great Britain.* London: H. Clowes & Son.
1887   *The Health of Nations,* vols. I and II. London: Longmans, Green and Co.

Churchman, C. West.
1968   *The Systems Approach.* New York: Dell.

Dubos, Rene.
1959   *Mirage of Health.* New York: Doubleday & Co.

Dhul, Leonard J.
1975   "The Process of Re-creation: The Health of the 'I' and the 'Us.' " Berkeley: University of California, Health and Medical Sciences.

Edelstein, Ludwig.
1967   *Ancient Medicine: Selected Papers of Ludwig Edelstein.* O. Temkin and C. L. Temkin, eds. Baltimore: Johns Hopkins.

Ehrenreich, John and Ehrenreich, Barbara.
1970   *The American Health Empire.* New York: Random House.
1974   "Health Care and Social Control," *Social Policy* 5:26-40.

Freidson, Eliot.
1970   *Profession of Medicine.* New York: Dodd, Mead.

Fuchs, Victor.
1966   "The Contribution of Health Services to the American Economy," *Milbank Memorial Fund Quarterly* 44(Part 2): 65:101.

Haberle, Rudolf.
1951   *Social Movements: An Introduction to Political Sociology.* New York: Appleton-Century-Crofts.

Hayes-Bautista, David E.
1976   "Deviant Delivery Systems." Paper presented at Conference on National Health Policy Issues, sponsored by the Western Consortium for Continuing Education for the Health Professions, San Francisco.

Kroeger, Gertrud.
1937   *The Concept of Social Medicine.* Chicago: Julius Rosenwald Fund.

Lynn, Walter R.
1969   "Systems Approach to Public Health," in Kilbourne and Smillie, eds., *Human Ecology and Public Health.* New York: Macmillan.

Parson, Talcott.
1951   *The Social System.* New York: Free Press.

Rosen, George.
1974   *From Medical Police to Social Medicine.* New York: Neale Watson.

Shattuck, Lemuel.
1948   *Report of the Sanitary Commission of Massachusetts, 1850.* Cambridge: Harvard University.

Simon, Harold.
1961   "Ideas, Germs and Society," *Stanford Medical Bulletin.* August.

Veatch, Robert M.
1973   "The Medical Model: Its Nature and Problems," *The Hastings Center Studies* 1 (3):58-76.

Winkelstein, Warren.
1972   "Epidemiological Considerations Underlying the Allocation of Health and Disease Care Resources," *International Journal of Epidemiology* 1 (1):69-74.

Measuring and Evaluating Hospital and Medical Care*

Avedis Donabedian

I have been asked to speak to you briefly about what I consider "the most serious problem in evaluating hospital and medical care, primarily focusing on inpatient treatment." This means that I must take a negative view, emphasizing how far short we are of our goal rather than extolling the considerable progress we may have made. Further, since the entire proceedings of this conference are within the context of professional responsibility for the quality of health care, I shall view the subject primarily from the standpoint of policy and action rather than of research.

At the outset, please note that my assignment is to speak about "the most serious *problem*" — in the singular, not the plural. "Surely," I thought when I first read this curious formulation, "this must be an error in typing. The problems are legion, and all are important; how could I single out one as the most serious?" And yet, strangely enough, there is one such problem that is the very root of all of our other difficulties, and it is this: we attempt to pass judgment on what we do not understand, or understand very imperfectly, at best. Everything I shall say from here on will be a variation on this central theme.

Ask an individual to talk about quality health care and you are likely to get a catalogue of platitudes. Ask two people and you will probably get an argument. Ask three, and you will probably have chaos. The reason is that each, like the proverbial blind men, has some different portion of the elephant in his hand.

Let me illustrate the problem by first showing you a visual approximation of the nature of the beast (see accompanying figure). It does not show great understanding that I have reduced the "elephant" to a cube. At least it is a solid; it is a beginning!

Note that one side of the cube shows several definitions of health, or extensions of a single definition; namely, physical-physiological, psychological, and social function. These are merely illustrative and are meant to show that our concept of quality — and, consequently, our criteria, our standards, and our measures — depend on how we define health and our responsibility for it.

On another side of the cube are illustrative steps indicating larger and more complex aggregations of the instrumentalities that provide care: the individual practitioner, groups of providers, and the system of care. This

From *Bulletin of the New York Academy of Medicine*, Vol. 52, No. 1, January 1976. By permission of the author and publisher.
*Presented in a panel, A Discussion of Methods, as part of the 1975 Annual Health Conference of the New York Academy of Medicine, *The Professional Responsibility for the Quality of Care*, held April 24 and 25, 1975.

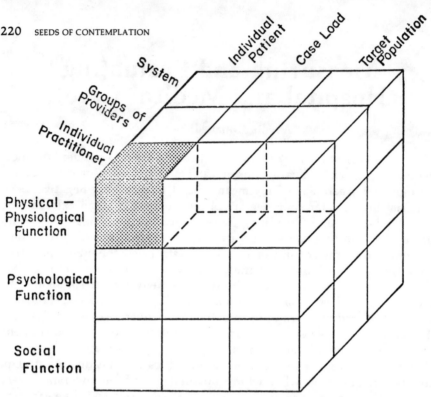

Schematic of frame of reference in simplified form.

suggests that beyond the most elementary level it becomes necessary to introduce into the criteria and measures of quality the joint contributions of more than one profession, as well as the attributes of continuity and coordination.

On the third side of the cube are steps in the aggregation of the client: individual patient, case load, and target population. The figure implies two separate notions: the distinction between patient and person and the distinction between an individual and an aggregate. Why should we make these distinctions? Because if our concern is with people as well as patients the concept of quality must include the attribute of access to care. Similarly, if our concern is for the aggregate as well as for the individual, our concept of quality must be broadened to include considerations of optimum allocation, given our necessarily limited resources. The allocation of resources is not simply a problem for those who make policy at the community level; it confronts every practitioner every moment of every day. Each practitioner is responsible for a case load of patients or a population of clients, and he must decide how to use his most precious resources — the practitioner's own time, attention, and concern — so as to serve best not only each patient singly, but all those who look to the practitioner for care.

Some additional concepts are illustrated by this cubic figure. First, it is likely that these three aspects do not exhaust the dimensions of quality. The reality is much more complex. Second, it becomes clear that almost all of our concern for quality has, so far, focused on only a small part of the figure: that representing the management of physical-physiological pathology in individual patients by individual practitioners, usually physicians. The immediate reaction to this observation is that we must expand the scope of our concern. But this cannot be done unilaterally or capriciously; some fundamental questions of professional domain and professional responsibility are at issue. In the most general terms, we cannot hold health practitioners responsible for that over which they have no control and we may not wish to expand their domain of control simply to achieve more conceptually satisfying definitions or estimates of the quality of care. However, it is not unreasonable to expect a practitioner to concern himself with the social and psychological concomitants of illness or to judge him by the manner in which he manages his entire case load of patients. Similarly, it is not unreasonable to expect a hospital to add to its concerns that of the aggregate effects of all the services that it offers. Finally, when a program, insititution, or individual practitioner is responsible for an enrolled population, the care of that entire population rather than of the subset of patients it generates must become the basis for judgment.

All of these extensions in the scope of our concern for quality are not unreasonable; yet, consider what horrendous difficulties they must create. We who are unable to decide how best to assess the quality of the technical management of physical-physiological illness shall be required, first, to determine criteria and standards for social and psychological management and, second, to resolve the ethical dilemmas of reconciling the interests of the individual patient with those of the collectivity — the heart of resource allocation. But we have no choice. We must venture forth.

From this prospect, which some will consider a challenge and others an unwarranted imposition, I shall turn to the more familiar realm of the technical management of physical-physiological illness.

The Health Insurance Plan of Greater New York pioneered in the study of the quality of medical care. In a paper which describes some of its work,[1] Henry Makover summarizes its principles by quoting from an editorial which appeared in the Lancet.[2]

> The other day an experienced physician was asked what criteria he would apply in judging the efficiency of a hospital; what relative importance he would attach to the qualifications of the staff, the ratio of beds to nurses, the adequacy of special departments, the catering, the facilities for reablement, and the various other items on which inspecting authorities commonly make notes. He replied, "I should not inquire into any of these things. I should simply go into the wards, select six patients, and find out precisely what had been done for them, and the care that they had received, since the day of their admission." This wise answer has implications beyond even the hospital services, for it embodies the truth that any kind of machinery, however ingenious, is but a means to an end.

Subsequent work at the Columbia University School of Public Health and Administrative Medicine under the leadership of Dr. Mildred Morehead was in this same tradition, except that almost exclusive reliance had to be placed on the medical record with all its recognized limitations as a source of information.[3][4] This deficiency — which could be rectified only in part by interviewing the attending physicians — was counterbalanced by the soundness of the basic idea of this study: that the judgment of quality in this context must depend on a complete assessment of the total care of a patient who presents as a problem for diagnosis and management, and that this assessment must reflect the best judgment of a mature and skilled physician charged with reviewing each case. Unfortunately, in hands less skillful than Dr. Morehead's the reliability of such judgments was found to be so low that the entire procedure has fallen into disrepute.

An alternative method that has been proposed originated in the pioneering work of Paul Lembeke. He devised what he called a "scientific method," which purported to remove the subjective element in assessments of quality by explicitly specifying the criteria by which judgments were to be made.[5] Subsequently, a similar approach was rediscovered independently by Beverly Payne;[6] it was tested in its most developed form in a study of hospital and ambulatory care in Hawaii.[7] The "criteria approach," as this method has come to be called, has since received such wide recognition that it has earned a central position in the projected nationwide system of Professional Standards Review Organizations. The sets of criteria that this system will generate presumably will stand as concrete embodiments, if not of quality care, at least of acceptable care. It is this concreteness and specificity that render the criteria approach so attractive. It adapts readily to the computer and the management of mass data. The judgments which it yields are likely to be highly replicable. What is at issue is their validity.

In assessing the validity of this approach we recognize that we are dealing with a generality. No doubt, the lists of criteria do vary in structure and content and may be put to different uses. For example, the method originally described by Lembeke was applied only to specified surgical operations and used only to judge whether the operation was to be considered justified or criticized, based on the evidence at hand. Even then, the judgment was further tempered by accepting the performance of teaching hospitals as the standard. By analogy, one might expect that the criteria would yield reasonably valid judgments as to the necessity for admission and readiness for discharge, although this has not been proved. But do the criteria, as currently designed, adequately represent the quality of care as more richly conceived? I shall argue that they do not and most probably cannot do so. Some of the shortcomings I shall mention can be remedied by a better designed program, but others are so basic that they call for a totally different approach.

All methods of assessment that begin with a sample of hospital records selected according to the primary discharge diagnosis or operative procedure share a number of defects. First, the sample excludes all cases that should have been so diagnosed or operated on in that manner, but were not. Thus a whole slice of performance remains totally in the dark. Second, there is considerable doubt that the performance of a physician or institution is so homogenous that a selection of diagnostic categories which is not a probability sample can stand for the total case load of that physician or institution.[8] Recent evidence based on a performance index using the criteria approach has shown generally low correlations in the performance of the same physicians across diagnostic categories.[9] Finally, in all instances the validity of these judgments is contingent upon the completeness and accuracy — if not the truthfulness — of the material in the record. While it is true that hospital practice and recording are correlated, the level of correlation appears to be low.[10] [11] Even if this correlation were high, the hospital record ordinarily would have little or no information about two important segments of care: those prior and subsequent to hospitalization.

Some additional deficiencies are particularly relevant to the criteria approach as ordinarily designed and implemented. To begin with, no account is taken of the presence of diagnoses additional to the primary one which may influence management — unless we assume that in large samples the presence and influence of such additional diagnoses tends to become comparable. Similarly, no account is taken of redundancy and wastefulness in management, whether in diagnostic investigation or treatment. The emphasis on justification of admission and readiness for discharge is an exception to this general observation. However, even here some important deficiencies may intrude. For example, if the criterion is readiness for discharge without attention to average length of stay, one could lose sight of how long it takes to become fit to leave the hospital and why. In considering the appropriateness of admission, it is unusual to ask some questions that should be fundamental to an assessment of quality: Could the disease have been prevented in the first place? Has hospitalization become necessary in part because of prior mismanagement?[12]

Closer to the assessment of hospital care itself, it is very unusual for those using the criteria approach to pass judgment on the accuracy of the diagnosis for discharge, the need for surgical intervention, or the choice of a particular operation. These are generally taken as given and attention is focused on whether the record of prior management includes the minimum set of activities that corresponds to these diagnoses or interventions — no matter what else has been done, how circuitous the path, or how proper the final destination. Strictly speaking, this is a test of internal consistency, an attribute which is at least one step removed from the quality of performance.

Assuming the diagnosis for discharge to be accurate and the minimum set of criteria to be relevant, further difficulties arise in constructing an over-all measure of performance which requires a summation of component subparts. It is usual to assume equal weights for all the items. Even when differential weights are assigned, as in the most recent work of Payne, it is not clear on what basis this is done.[7] It is seldom, if ever, recognized that the process of management consists of highly interactive parts and that when certain key elements are lacking the care as a whole must be judged as poor no matter how many of the other criteria elements have been performed and recorded.

This is the core of the problem. Clinical management is a complex process of making diagnostic and therapeutic decisions. It is based on factual knowledge, but requires something additional which we recognize as clinical judgment — which is at the heart of technical quality. Clinical judgment involves deciding what alternatives to consider in diagnosis and therapy, how far to go in seeking what degree of certainty, what means to use, what risks to incur relative to what probability of success in seeking how large a benefit, when to act, and when to watchfully wait. What a far cry from the sterotyped behavior embodied in the lists of criteria — which so easily can become distorted into an indiscriminate assemblage of the elements of care until they are almost a caricature of clinical judgment rather than its true representation. No wonder that physicians are almost intuitively repelled by the very thought of being judged by these.

When, then, is to be done? Shall we, because clinical judgment is so complex and elusive to measure, give up all thought of assessing the quality of care? This certainly is not my conclusion. We need to further develop and refine the criteria so that they become a realistic model of the clinical process rather than a distortion. But we cannot do this unless we gain a greater understanding of the clinical process itself through more rigorous conceptual and empirical work. I repeat, we cannot evaluate in a defensible manner what we do not clearly understand, and we now only dimly perceive the attributes of clinical judgment. We urgently need basic research on the clinical process itself, so that we can delineate the different pathways it can take and the costs and benefits of each — both monetary and nonmonetary — to the individual and to society. In the pursuit of this end we may learn from what is already known about problem-solving and trouble-shooting behavior in general[13] and about clinical decision-making in particular.[14]

But what are we to do as we await the advent of the more perfect instrument? First, it is salutary to remember that many deficiencies in care are so gross that no refinement is necessary to detect them: they fairly leap at you, provided you care to look. Second, the criteria approach can be modified to meet many of the criticisms that we have leveled against it. In particular, the use of these criteria must be judicious and prudent, with full cognizance of their many limitations as arbiters of quality. It would be tragic to yield to the temptation to use them primarily as devices to police and punish. Third, any system of quality assessment and assurance must include information about all the important aspects of care obtained from a variety of sources. Among the most important of these, as the Committee on the Standardization of Hospitals recommended more than 60 years ago,[15] is information about proximate and remote end results of care. Finally, we must remember that until a more objective method is devised the ultimate arbiter of the quality of clinical management must remain the judgment of our wisest and most competent colleagues when they are given all the facts of each case. We shall be unable to improve upon this until the bases for judgment are made explicit and measurable and are subjected to wider professional and social validation.

FOOTNOTES

1. Makover, H.B.: The quality of medical care: Methodology of survey of medical groups associated with the Health Insurance Plan of Greater New York. *Amer. J. Public Health 41*: 824-32, 1951 (see esp. pp. 825 and 826).
2. Mechanism and purpose. Editorial. *Lancet 1*:27-28, 1950.
3. Ehrlich, J., Morehead, M.A., and Trussell, R.E.: *The Quantity, Quality and Costs of Medical and Hospital Care Secured by a Sample of Teamster Families in the New York Area.* Monograph. New York, Columbia University School of Public Health and Administrative Medicine, 1962.
4. Morehead, M.A., Donaldson, R.S., Sanderson, S., and Burt, F.: *A Study of the Quality of Hospital Care Secured by a Sample of Teamster Family Members in New York City.* Monograph. New York, Columbia University School of Public Health and Administrative Medicine, 1964.
5. Lembcke, P.A.: Medical auditing by scientific methods. *J.A.M.A. 162*:646-55, 1956.
6. Payne, B.C.: Continued evolution of a system of medical care appraisal. *J.A.M.A. 20*:536-40, 1967.
7. Payne, B.C. and Lyons, T.F.: *Method of Evaluating and Improving Personal Medical Care Quality: Episode of Illness Study.* Ann Arbor, Mich., The University of Michigan School of Medicine, 1972.
8. Donabedian, A.: *A Guide to Medical Care Administration, Volume II: Medical Care Appraisal — Quality and Utilization.* New York, Amer. Public Health Ass. Inc., 1969, pp. 53-56.
9. Lyons, T.F. and Payne, B.C.: Interdiagnosis relationships of physician performance measures. *Med. Care 12*:369-74, 1974.
10. Rosenfeld, L. S.: Quality of medical care in hospitals. *Amer. J. Public Health 47*:856-65, 1957.
11. Lyons, T.F. and Payne, B.C.: The relationship of physicians' medical recording performance to their medical care performance. *Med. Care 12*:714-20, 1974.
12. These aspects of performance were pointed out to me by Paul M. Gertman, Director, Health Services Research and Development Program, Boston University Medical Center, Boston, Mass.
13. Donabedian, A.: Evaluating the Quality of Medical Care. *Milbank Mem. Fund Quart. 44*:166-203, 1966, Part 2 (see esp. pp. 194-195 and references 63-70).
14. Barnoon, S. and Wolfe, H.: *Measuring the Effectiveness of Medical Decisions: An Operations Research Approach.* Springfield, Ill., Thomas, 1972.
15. Committee on Standardization of Hospitals. End result record system suggested by the Committee on Standardization of Hospitals. *Surg. Gynec. Obstet.* (Suppl.) *18*:9-12, 1914.

Medical Nemesis

Ivan Illich

Within the last decade medical professional practice has become a major threat to health. Depression, infection, disability, dysfunction, and other specific iatrogenic diseases now cause more suffering than all accidents from traffic or industry. Beyond this, medical practice sponsors sickness by the reinforcement of a morbid society which not only industrially preserves its defectives but breeds the therapist's client in a cybernetic way. Finally, the so-called health-professions have an indirect sickening power — a structurally health-denying effect. I want to focus on this last syndrome, which I designate as medical Nemesis. By transforming pain, illness, and death from a personal challenge into a technical problem, medical practice expropriates the potential of people to deal with their human condition in an autonomous way and becomes the source of a new kind of un-health.

Much suffering has always been man-made: history is the record of enslavement and exploitation. It tells of war, and of the pillage, famine, and pestilence which come in its wake. War between commonwealths and classes has so far been the main planned agency of man-made misery. Thus, man is the only animal whose evolution has been conditioned by adaptation on two fronts. If he did not succumb to the elements, he had to cope with use and abuse by others of his kind. He replaced instincts by character and culture, to be capable of this struggle on two frontiers. A third frontier of possible doom has been recognised since Homer; but common mortals were considered immune to its threat. Nemesis, the Greek name for the awe which loomed from this third direction, was the fate of a few heroes who had fallen prey to the envy of the gods. The common man grew up and perished in a struggle with Nature and neighbour. Only the élite would challenge the thresholds set by Nature for man.

Prometheus was not Everyman, but a deviant. Driven by Pleonexia, or radical greed, he trespassed the boundaries of the human condition. In hubris or measureless presumption, he brought fire from heaven, and thereby brought Nemesis on himself. He was put into irons on a Caucasian rock. A vulture preys at his innards, and heartlessly healing gods keep him alive by regrafting his liver each night. The encounter with Nemesis made the classical hero an immortal reminder of inescapable cosmic retaliation. He becomes a subject for epic tragedy, but certainly not a model for everyday aspiration. Now Nemesis has become endemic; it is the backlash of progress. Paradoxically, it has spread as far and as wide as the franchise, schooling, mechanical acceleration, and medical care. Everyman has fallen

From *The Lancet*, Vol. I, No. 7863, May 11, 1974. By permission of the author and publisher. This article was the author's first draft for a book that was published under the title *Medical Nemesis — The Limits To Medicine* by Pantheon, New York, 1976 and by M. Boyars, London, 1976.

prey to the envy of the gods. If the species is to survive it can do so only by learning to cope in this third group.

Industrial Nemesis

Most man-made misery is now the byproduct of enterprises which were originally designed to protect the common man in his struggle with the inclemency of the environment and against wanton injustices inflicted by the élite. The main source of pain, disability, and death is now an engineered — albeit non-intentional — harassment. The prevailing ailments, helplessness and injustice, are now the side-effects of strategies for progress. Nemesis is now so prevalent that it is readily mistaken for part of the human condition. The desperate disability of contemporary man to envisage an alternative to the industrial aggression on the human condition is an integral part of the curse from which he suffers. Progress has come with a vengeance which cannot be called a price. The down payment was on the label and can be stated in measurable terms. The instalments accrue under forms of suffering which exceed the notion of "pain."

At some point in the expansion of our major institutions their clients begin to pay a higher price every day for their continued consumption, in spite of the evidence that they will inevitably suffer more. At this point in development the prevalent behaviour of society corresponds to that traditionally recognised in addicts. Declining returns pale in comparison with marginally increasing disutilities. *Homo economicus* turns into *Homo religiosus*. His expectations become heroic. The vengeance of economic development not only outweighs the price at which this vengeance was purchased; it also outweighs the compound tort done by Nature and neighbours. Classical Nemesis was punishment for the rash abuse of a privilege. Industrialised Nemesis is retribution for dutiful participation in society.

War and hunger, pestilence and sudden death, torture and madness remain man's companions, but they are now shaped into a new *Gestalt* by the Nemesis overarching them. The greater the economic progress of any community, the greater the part played by industrial Nemesis in the pain, discrimination, and death suffered by its members. Therefore, it seems that the disciplined study of the distinctive character of Nemesis ought to be the key theme for research amongst those who are concerned with health care, healing, and consoling.

Tantalus

Medical Nemesis is but one aspect of the more general "counter-intuitive misadventures" characteristic of industrial society. It is the monstrous outcome of a very specific dream of reason — namely, "tantalising" hubris. Tantalus was a famous king whom the gods invited to Olympus to share one of their meals. He purloined Ambrosia, the divine potion which gave the gods unending life. For punishment, he was made immortal in Hades and condemned to suffer unending thirst and hunger. When he bows towards the river in which he stands, the water recedes, and when he reaches for the fruit above his head the branches move out of his reach. Ethologists might say that Hygienic Nemesis has programmed him for compulsory counter-intuitive behaviour. Craving for Ambrosia has now spread to the common mortal. Scientific and political optimism have combined to propagate the addiction. To sustain it, the priesthood of Tantalus has organised itself, offering unlimited medical improvement of human health. The members of this guild pass themselves off as disciples of healing Asklepios, while in fact they peddle Ambrosia. People demand of them that life be improved, prolonged, rendered compatible with machines, and capable of surviving all modes of acceleration, distortion, and stress. As a result, health has become scarce to the degree to which the common man makes health depend upon the consumption of Ambrosia.

Culture and Health

Mankind evolved only because each of its individuals came into existence protected by various visible and invisible cocoons. Each one knew the womb from which he had come, and oriented himself by the stars under which he was born. To be human and to become human, the individual of our species has to find his destiny in his unique struggle with Nature and neighbour. He is on his own in the struggle, but the weapons and the rules and the style are given to him by the culture in which he grew up. Each culture is the sum of rules with which the individual could come to terms with pain, sickness, and death — could interpret them and practice compassion amongst others faced by the same threats. Each culture set the myth, the rituals, the taboos, and the ethical standards needed to deal with the fragility of life — to explain the reason for pain, the dignity of the sick, and the role of dying or death.

Cosmopolitan medical civilisation denies the need for man's acceptance of these evils. Medical civilisation is planned and organised to kill pain, to eliminate sickness, and to struggle against death. These are new goals, which have never before been guidelines for social life and which are antithetic to every one of the cultures with which medical civilisation meets when it is dumped on the so-called poor as part and parcel of their economic progress.

The health-denying effect of medical civilisation is thus equally powerful in rich and in poor countries, even though the latter are often spared some of its more sinister sides.

The Killing of Pain

For an experience to be pain in the full sense, it must fit into a culture. Precisely because each culture provides a mode for suffering, culture is a particular form of health. The act of suffering is shaped by culture into a question which can be stated and shared.

Medical civilisation replaces the culturally determined competence in suffering with a growing demand by each individual for the institutional management of his pain. A myriad of different feelings, each expressing some kind of fortitude, are homogenised into the political pressure of anaesthesia consumers. Pain becomes an item on a list of complaints. As a result, a new kind of horror emerges. Conceptually it is still pain, but the impact on our emotions of this valueless, opaque, and impersonal hurt is something quite new.

In this way, pain has come to pose only a technical question for industrial man — what do I need to get in order to have my pain managed or killed? If the pain continues, the fault is not with the universe, God, my sins, or the devil, but with the medical system. Suffering is an expression of consumer demand for increased medical outputs. By becoming unnecessary, pain has become unbearable. With this attitude, it now seems rational to flee pain rather than to face it, even at the cost of addiction. It also seems reasonable to eliminate pain, even at the cost of health. It seems enlightened to deny legitimacy to all non-technical issues which pain raises, even at the cost of disarming the victims of residual pain. For a while it can be argued that the total pain anaesthetised in a society is greater than the totality of pain newly generated. But at some point, rising marginal disutilities set in. The new suffering is not only unmanageable, but it has lost its referential character. It has become meaningless, questionless torture. Only the recovery of the will and ability to suffer can restore health into pain.

The Elimination of Sickness

Medical interventions have not affected total mortality-rates: at best they have shifted survival from one segment of the population to another. Dramatic changes in the nature of disease afflicting Western societies during the last 100 years are well documented. First industrialisation exacerbated infections, which then subsided. Tuberculosis peaked over a 50-75-year period and declined before either the tubercle bacillus had been discovered or anti-tuberculous programmes had been initiated. It was replaced in Britain and the U.S. by major malnutrition syndromes — rickets and pellagra — which peaked and declined, to be replaced by disease of early childhood, which in turn gave way to duodenal ulcers in young men. When that declined the modern epidemics took their toll — coronary heart-disease, hypertension, cancer, arthritis, diabetes, and mental disorders. At least in the U.S., death-rates from hypertensive heart-disease seem to be declining. Despite intensive research no connection between these changes in disease patterns can be attributed to the professional practice of medicine.

Neither decline in any of the major epidemics of killing diseases, nor major changes in the age structure of the population, nor falling and rising absenteeism at the workbench have been significantly related to sick care — even to immunisation. Medical services deserve neither credit for longevity nor blame for the threatening population pressure.

Longevity owes much more to the railroad and to the synthesis of fertilisers and insecticides than it owes to new drugs and syringes. Professional practice is both ineffective and increasingly sought out. This technically unwarranted rise of medical prestige can only be explained as a magical ritual for the achievement of goals which are beyond technical and political reach. It can be countered only through legislation and political action which favours the deprofessionalisation of health care.

The overwhelming majority of modern diagnostic and therapeutic interventions which demonstrably do more good than harm have two characteristics: the material resources for them are extremely cheap, and they can be packaged and designed for self-use or application by family members. The price of technology that is significantly health-furthering or curative in Canadian medicine is so low that the resources now squandered in India on modern medicine would suffice to make it available in the entire sub-continent. On the other hand, the skills needed for the application of the most generally used diagnostic and therapeutic aids are so simple that the careful observation of instruction by people who personally care would guarantee more effective and responsible use than medical practice can provide.

The deprofessionalisation of medicine does not imply and should not be read as implying negation of specialised healers, of competence, of mutual criticism, or of public control. It does imply a bias against mystification, against transnational dominance of one orthodox view, against disbarment of healers chosen by their patients but not certified by the guild. The deprofessionalisation of medicine does not mean denial of public funds for curative purposes, it does mean a bias against the disbursement of any such funds under the prescription and control of guild-members, rather than under the control of the consumer. Deprofessionalisation does not mean the elimination of modern medicine, nor obstacles to the invention of new ones, nor necessarily the return to ancient programmes, rituals, and devices. It means that no professional shall have the power to lavish on any one of his patients a package of curative resources larger than that which any other could claim on his own. Finally, the deprofessionalisation of medicine does not mean disregard for the special needs which people manifest at special moments of their lives; when they are born, break a leg, marry, give birth, become crippled, or face death. It only means that people have a right to live in an environment which is hospitable to them at such high points of experience.

The Struggle Against Death

The ultimate effect of medical Nemesis is the expropriation of death. In every society the image of death is the culturally conditioned anticipation of an uncertain date. This anticipation determines a series of behavioural norms during life and the structure of certain institutions.

Wherever modern medical civilisation has penetrated a traditional medical culture, a novel cultural ideal of death has been fostered. The new ideal spreads by means of technology and the professional ethos which corresponds to it.

In primitive societies death is always conceived as the intervention of an actor — an enemy, a witch, an ancestor, or a god. The Christian and the Islamic Middle Ages saw in each death the hand of God. Western death had no face until about 1420. The Western ideal of death which comes to all equally from natural causes is of quite recent origin. Only during the autumn of the Middle Ages death appears as a skeleton with power in its own right. Only during the 16th century, as an answer European peoples developed the "arte and crafte to knowe ye Will to Dye." For the next three centuries peasant and noble, priest and whore, prepared themselves throughout life to preside at their own death. Foul death, bitter death, became the end rather than the goal of living. The idea that natural death should come only in healthy old age appeared only in the 18th century as a class-specific phenomenon of the bourgeois. The demand that doctors struggle against death and keep valetudinarians healthy has nothing to do with their ability to provide such service: Ariès has shown that the costly attempts to prolong life appear at first only among bankers whose power is compounded by the years they spend at a desk.

We cannot fully understand contemporary social organisation unless we see in it a multi-faceted exorcism of all forms of evil death. Our major institutions constitute a gigantic defence programme waged on behalf of "humanity" against all those people who can be associated with what is currently conceived of as death-dealing social injustice. Not only medical agencies, but welfare, international relief, and development programmes are enlisted in this struggle. Ideological bureaucracies of all colours join the crusade. Even war has been used to justify the defeat of those who are blamed for wanton tolerance of sickness and death. Producing "natural death" for all men is at the point of becoming an ultimate justification for social control. Under the influence of medical rituals contemporary death is again the rationale for a witch-hunt.

Conclusion

Rising irreparable damage accompanies industrial expansion in all sectors. In medicine these damages appear as iatrogenesis. Iatrogenesis can be direct, when pain, sickness, and death result from medical care; or it can be indirect, when health policies reinforce an industrial organisation which generates ill-health: it can be structural when medically sponsored behaviour and delusion restrict the vital autonomy of people by under-mining their competence in growing up, caring, ageing; or when it nullifies the personal challenge arising from their pain, disability, and anguish.

Most of the remedies proposed to reduce iatrogenesis are engineering interventions. They are therapeutically designed in their approach to the individual, the group, the institution, or the environment. These so-called remedies generate second-order iatrogenic ills by creating a new prejudice against the autonomy of the citizen.

The most profound iatrogenic effects of the medical technostructure result from its non-technical social functions. The sickening technical and non-technical consequences of the institutionalisation of medicine coalesce to generate a new kind of suffering — anaesthetised and solitary survival in a world-wide hospital ward.

Medical Nemesis cannot be operationally verified. Much less can it be measured. The intensity with which it is experienced depends on the independence, vitality, and relatedness of each individual. As a theoretical concept it is one component in a broad theory to explain the anomalies plaguing health-care systems in our day. It is a district aspect of an even more general phenomenon which I have called industrial Nemesis, the backlash of institutionally structured industrial hubris. This hubris consists of a disregard for the boundaries within which the human phenomenon remains viable. Current research is overwhelmingly oriented towards unattainable "breakthroughs." What I have called counterfoil research is the disciplined analysis of the levels at which such reverberations must inevitably damage man.

The perception of enveloping Nemesis leads to a social choice. Either the natural boundaries of human endeavour are estimated, recognised, and translated into politically determined limits, or the alternative to extinction is compulsory survival in a planned and engineered Hell.

In several nations the public is ready for a review of its health-care system. The frustrations which have become manifest from private-enterprise systems and from socialised care have come to resemble each other frighteningly. The differences between the annoyances of the Russian, French, Americans, and English have become trivial. There is a serious danger that these evaluations will be performed within the coordinates set by post-cartesian illusions. In rich and poor countries the demand for reform of national health care is dominated by demands for equitable access to the wares of the guild, professional expansion and sub-professionalisation, and for more truth in the advertising of progress and lay-control of the temple of Tantalus. The public discussion of the health crisis could easily be used to channel even more power, prestige, and money to biomedical engineers and designers.

There is still time in the next few years to avoid a debate which would reinforce a frustrating system. The coming debate can be reoriented by making medical Nemesis the central issue. The explanation of Nemesis requires simultaneous assessment of both the technical and the non-technical side of medicine — and must focus on it as both industry and religion. The indictment of medicine as a form of institutional hubris exposes precisely those personal illusions which make the critic dependent on the health care.

The perception and comprehension of Nemesis has therefore the power of leading us to policies which could break the magic circle of complaints which now reinforce the dependence of the plaintiff on the health engineering and planning agencies whom he sues. Recognition of Nemesis can provide the catharsis to prepare for a non-violent revolution in our attitudes towards evil and pain. The alternative to a war against these ills is the search for the peace of the strong.

Health designates a process of adaptation. It is not the result of instinct, but of autonomous and live reaction to an experienced reality. It designates the ability to adapt to changing environments, to growing up and to ageing, to healing when damaged, to suffering and to the peaceful expectation of death. Health embraces the future as well, and therefore includes anguish and the inner resource to live with it.

Man's consciously lived fragility, individuality, and relatedness make the experience of pain, of sickness, and of death an integral part of his life. The ability to cope with this trio in autonomy is fundamental to his health. To the degree to which he becomes dependent on the management of his intimacy he renounces his autonomy and his health *must* decline. The true miracle of modern medicine is diabolical. It consists of making not only individuals but whole populations survive on inhumanly low levels of personal health. That health should decline with increasing health-service delivery is unforeseen only by the health manager, precisely because his strategies are the result of his blindness to the inalienability of health.

The level of public health corresponds to the degree to which the means and responsibility for coping with illness are distributed amongst the total population. This ability to cope can be enhanced but never replaced by medical intervention in the lives of people or the hygienic characteristics of the environment. That society which can reduce professional inter-vention to the minimum will provide the best conditions for health. The greater the potential for autonomous adaptation to self and to others and to the environment, the less management of adaptation will be needed or tolerated.

The recovery of health attitude towards sickness is neither Luddite nor Romantic nor Utopian: it is a guiding ideal which will never be fully achieved, which can be achieved with modern devices as never before in history, and which must orient politics to avoid encroaching Nemesis.